The
Food-Mood
Solution

The
Food-Mood
Solution

All-Natural Ways to Banish Anxiety, Depression, Anger, Stress, Overeating, and Alcohol and Drug Problems— and Feel Good Again

JACK CHALLEM

Foreword by Melvyn R. Werbach, M.D.

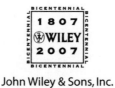

BICENTENNIAL
1807
WILEY
2007
BICENTENNIAL

John Wiley & Sons, Inc.

Published by John Wiley & Sons, Inc., Hoboken, New Jersey
Published simultaneously in Canada

Wiley Bicentennial Logo: Richard J. Pacifico

Design and composition by Navta Associates, Inc.

The information contained in this book is not intended to serve as a replacement for professional medical advice. Any use of the information in this book is at the reader's discretion. The author and the publisher specifically disclaim any and all liability arising directly or indirectly from the use or application of any information contained in this book. A health care professional should be consulted regarding your specific situation.

For general information about our other products and services, please contact our Customer Care Department within the United States at (800) 762-2974, outside the United States at (317) 572-3993 or fax (317) 572-4002.

Wiley also publishes its books in a variety of electronic formats. Some content that appears in print may not be available in electronic books. For more information about Wiley products, visit our web site at www.wiley.com.

Library of Congress Cataloging-in-Publication Data:
Challem, Jack.
  The food-mood solution : all-natural ways to banish anxiety, depression, anger, stress,
overeating, and alcohol and drug problems / Jack Challem ; foreword by Melvyn R. Werbach.
      p. cm.
  Includes bibliographical references and index.
  ISBN 978-0-471-75610-1 (cloth)
  1. Mental health—Nutritional aspects. 2. Mood (Psychology)—Nutritional aspects.
3. Nutritionally induced diseases. I. Title.
  RC455.4.N8C44 2007
  616.89'0654—dc22

                                                                    2006021036

Printed in the United States of America

10 9 8 7 6 5 4 3 2 1

For Helen

CONTENTS

FOREWORD

The evidence for a body-mind connection in health and disease is overwhelming. Our bodies and minds are deeply interconnected and mutually dependent. As but one example, we've long known that optimists tend to live healthier and longer lives compared with pessimists, and that stress and depression increase our risk of disease. Why is this? When we're happy, our bodies and minds make numerous health-promoting chemicals. When we're sad or angry, our bodies and minds make many disease-promoting chemicals.

As self-evident as a unified, integrated approach to healing may be, we are just now emerging from many centuries in which the body and the mind were treated as if they were totally separate entities. How misguided this dichotomy has been! The same nourishing blood that flows through our hearts also feeds our brains. Although Western medicine is slowly awakening to integrative concepts, it still suffers from the remnants of its body-*or*-mind heritage. The training of mental health practitioners is frequently restricted to either psychological or physical approaches to treatment. All too often, a person's mental health, emotional feelings, and behavior continue to be treated as if they have nothing to do with physical health.

It's not that a purely psychological or a purely physical approach is wrong. The problem is that a limited approach will produce only limited results. The power of an integrative approach is that it weaves together multiple interventions, increasing the chances of improvement. An integrative approach to negative moods and behavior doesn't seek only a single cause. Rather, it usually identifies many intertwined causes.

Likewise, an integrative approach doesn't treat a problem in just one way. Rather, it treats the problem in as many ways as possible. Such multipronged treatments focus on methods that are safe, effective, easy to follow, and inexpensive.

So many self-help books offer "do this" or "take that" suggestions for improving moods, behavior, and relationships. These books provide some useful advice, but they frequently suffer from too limited a perspective. This tunnel vision ultimately fails the reader because it ignores so many potentially helpful approaches. Not surprisingly, the results of such narrow approaches are often disappointing.

In his latest book, *The Food-Mood Solution*, Jack Challem avoids these common pitfalls. He draws on his training as a sociologist and his experience in the field of nutrition to describe what could be called the body-mind-nutrition connection. What has nutrition got to do with moods and behavior? It is nutrition that feeds both body and mind. The food we eat supplies the biochemical basis for everything that happens (or should happen) in our bodies. Nutrients enable our bodies to turn genes on and off, to catalyze the tens of thousands of necessary chemical reactions that occur every second of every day, to enable the functioning of our heart and lungs and skin, and to make the many essential brain chemicals that influence our moods and behavior.

It is easy to consider nutrition the missing link in modern medicine, when it should rightfully be treated as the foundation of health. In my many years of psychiatric practice, I frequently found that different people with identical complaints responded to different treatments. These differences are related to individual variations in genetics, stress, lifestyle, and nutrition. I learned early on that nutrition was one of the most important aspects of an individual's health to consider, and that knowledge of how nutrition affected mood and behavior was often helpful—and sometimes crucial—to improving a patient's mental state. Dietary improvements and nutritional supplements relieved anxiety and depression by fostering biochemical changes that enhance mood. Sometimes they accomplished this by correcting a nutrient deficiency. Other times, nutrients accelerated specific biochemical healing reactions. In either case, nutrients consistently accomplished their results with far fewer adverse reactions than those caused by drugs.

Jack Challem's *The Food-Mood Solution* simply and succinctly describes the nutritional underpinnings of our neurotransmitters—brain chemicals, such as serotonin, that affect our moods and behavior. He recommends dietary changes and nutritional supplements to enhance production of appropriate neurotransmitters for people who feel angry, anxious, irritable, impulsive, distracted, depressed, or just plain moody. Yet, to his credit, Jack doesn't just give another set of nutrition prescriptions. He arms us with knowledge of how our modern lifestyle generates tremendous feelings of stress, and how the pressures of work and home disrupt healthy eating habits and moods. Jack also dispenses straightforward psychological and lifestyle advice and tips for resisting stress and mellowing even the most negative of moods.

The Food-Mood Solution unleashes the power of integrative healing into the world of self-help. One advantage of this book is that its advice is so direct, clear, and easy to apply. You will learn the basics of how your mood is modified by what you eat and, conversely, how your nutrition requirements are modified by your moods. Equally important, you will learn which specific lifestyle changes to make to help you move from negative feelings and moods toward a sense of greater contentment and calmness—that is, feeling better about yourself and the many good people in your life.

I'd like you to consider *The Food-Mood Solution* a manual for a happier, more satisfying life. Will you have to make some changes? Of course, you will, and that will take a little effort. But you will feel better so quickly and your outlook will be so much brighter that you will be motivated to make even greater changes in your life.

Melvyn R. Werbach, M.D.
Diplomate in Psychiatry, American Board of
Psychiatry and Neurology
Author, *Nutritional Influences on Mental Illness*
Associate Editor, *Alternative Therapies in Health and Medicine*

ACKNOWLEDGMENTS

This book is the synthesis of many different ideas and a wide range of research and applications. A great many people contributed to it by influencing my thinking over the years. In the realm of nutritional medicine, Abram Hoffer, M.D., Ph.D., and the late Hugh D. Riordan, M.D., played key roles in my opinions about nutrition and behavior. My conversations with William Walsh, Ph.D., Priscilla Slagle, M.D., and the late Theron Randolph, M.D., were also influential.

I owe a debt of gratitude to Ronald E. Hunninghake, M.D., of the Bright Spot for Health, in Wichita, Kansas, for his knowledge of medicine and biochemistry and his willingness to always explore ideas with me. I also want to thank Joy Weydert, M.D., for sharing some of her knowledge about the nutritional basis of neurotransmitters. Special thanks go to Loretta Kramer, an extraordinarily perceptive counselor, for her comments and insights.

I'd like to thank Jack Scovil, my literary agent, and Thomas Miller, my editor, for their continued support and contributions to the shaping of this book. I'd also like to acknowledge Mike Millard, Joan Miller, and Bill Thomson for helping me to refine some of the concepts in this book. In addition, I thank Kimberly Monroe-Hill and Patricia Waldygo for their exceptional editing.

Last but not least, I'd like to thank Helen Selwitschka, who came into my life in one of those rare examples of serendipity. Whether it was by chance, convergence, or fate, I appreciate what you've added to this book and to my life.

Introduction

A few people will raise their eyebrows when they hear that I've written a book about improving bad moods. I've certainly had my share of moods over the years, and, if you're like most people, you've had yours as well.

It's normal to develop a negative mood in response to difficult situations, especially those we have no control over. It's not normal, however, to be in a pissy mood most of the time. Nor is it normal to feel anxious, spacey, down, or extremely moody much of the time. Over the last few years, I've learned how to maintain more stable and upbeat moods. I may still get angry if someone intentionally tries to hurt me, but I now let go of that negative mood fairly quickly instead of letting it consume me.

If you look at people around you, the reality is pretty obvious: more and more of them are prickly, irritable, abrasive, and angry or have other mood and behavior problems. It's not just your imagination. A 2005 survey found that people believe that rude behavior is far more common than it was twenty or thirty years ago. Drivers honk their horns to punish the mistakes of other drivers. Office workers impatiently start boarding an elevator before others get off. Many people seethe in frustration while waiting in line at banks or supermarkets.

Some of us inflict our mood swings on employees and family members, and others seem hell-bent on physical violence. In 2006, police reports from across the country noted a surge in murders resulting from dumb and petty arguments, such as disagreeing over a dress, using the wrong soap dish, giving another person a dirty look, looking at someone's girlfriend the wrong way, or accidentally bumping into someone. The Philadelphia police commissioner was quoted in the *New York Times* as saying, "It's arguments—stupid arguments over stupid things."

Being as self-centered as we often are, we invariably blame everyone else when other people don't act the way we want them to. The situation reminds me of George Carlin's joke about drivers: if someone is going too fast, we think he's a maniac, and if she's going too slow, she's retarded. We're the only ones who are normal and balanced, right?

Jokes aside, you or someone you know may be guilty of the behavior I described. If you see yourself in what I've written, the good news is that this book can help you to improve your moods and deal with the inevitable stresses of life.

Our Society's Increasingly Negative Mood

Over the last twenty years, our society's mood as a whole has grown much worse. Argumentativeness, meanness, and unwillingness to compromise now pervade politics—but they're not restricted to politics. Who among us commutes and does not regularly encounter some form of meanness or recklessness on the part of other drivers—or is not guilty of it himself?

As an example, in the late 1980s, I moved to Beaverton, Oregon, and was immediately struck by the courtesy of drivers. This changed during a boom in the local high-tech economy, when thousands of people relocated from California and brought with them their notorious driving habits. The politeness I had experienced vanished in a sea of aggressive SUVs and BMWs.

Although drivers in some cities, such as New York and Los Angeles, are known for their aggressive habits, the same patterns began to appear in small towns and cities throughout the country. Drivers' muttering under their breath morphed into shouts, obscene gestures, road rage, and freeway shootings. The problem is not only with driving habits. There has been an epidemic of what I call "pissy mood syndrome." All too many people are in an irritable mood much of the time.

How Many People Have Bad Moods?

Just how common are our bad moods? Recent articles in the *Archives of General Psychiatry*, published by the American Medical Association, have pointed out that at least one of every two people will experience a serious mood or mental health problem at some time in his or her life.

One of every two people is a pretty sobering number, but other statistics from the same study are just as unsettling. Almost one in every three people will suffer from at least one serious bout of anxiety, including panic disorder, obsessive-compulsive disorder, phobia, social anxiety, and post-traumatic stress disorder. One in four people will have some sort of impulsive-control problem, such as explosive outbursts and defiant behavior. One in five people will suffer from serious depression or bipolar (manic-depressive) disorder. One in every eight people will abuse alcohol or drugs.

A separate study, also in the *Archives of General Psychiatry*, reported that slightly more than 9 percent of American adults currently have serious mood disorders, and another 11 percent have clear-cut anxiety disorders. These percentages add up to a frightening 42 million adults, equivalent to the combined populations of New York, Illinois, Oregon, Colorado, and Connecticut. Stuart C. Yudofsky, M.D., a psychiatry professor at the Baylor College of Medicine, Houston, has estimated that almost 15 percent of Americans have a personality disorder, which might include mood swings and instability, impulsiveness, or some sort of self-defeating or self-destructive behavior. Yudofsky has also estimated that another 15 to 30 percent of people have a family member, a friend, or a coworker with a serious personality disorder.

This high prevalence of mood and behavior disorders is disturbing enough, but the numbers may actually be even higher. If you have had one bout with a serious mood disorder, you are likely to have another. Furthermore, these studies reflect the number of people who have had problems serious enough to be flagged by doctors. If you're simply irritable, impulsive, anxious, depressed, angry, or physically aggressive—but are never diagnosed by a doctor or arrested by the police—you and millions of other people go through life below the medical and legal radar.

What Causes Bad Moods?

Our bad moods result from a variety of factors. We feel stressed at work, at home, and while commuting, and we feel as though we must do more in less time. Often, our bosses, our customers, and people who are closest to us simply don't understand how much pressure we're under, what we're trying to juggle, how hard we push ourselves, and how close we are to being totally fatigued. When we feel stressed and tired, we're more likely to be pushed closer to the edge.

Yet our bad moods also result from eating bad, or unhealthy, foods. In one study, researchers found that 80 percent of people with mood disorders knew that the foods they ate affected how they felt. Sugary foods and alcohol contributed to mood problems, whereas fish, vegetables, and fruit were associated with better moods. The translation: bad foods set the stage for bad moods, while good foods led to good moods.

What could food possibly have to do with our moods? The answer might surprise you. Nutrients provide the biological building blocks for brain chemicals called *neurotransmitters*, which affect how we think and feel. You probably know that when you work too hard to eat on time, your mood and energy levels likely suffer. When you don't eat enough high-quality *neuronutri-ents*—literally, "brain nutrients"—your body cannot make adequate amounts of mood-enhancing neurotransmitters.

> **Quick Tip**
>
> **What Is a Neuronutrient?**
> Neuronutrients are vitamins, minerals, and related nutrients that are needed to make neurotransmitters. Neurotransmitters, in turn, are the chemicals that control our moods.

The Nutrisocial Concept: Where Society and Eating Habits Intersect

The relationship between food and mood is far more complicated than the so-called Twinkie defense some lawyers have used in criminal trials.

(That is, "Junk foods made him do it.") Your body needs vitamins, protein, and other nutrients to make the brain chemicals that help you think clearly, maintain a good mood, and act in socially acceptable ways. I use the term *neuronutrients* to describe these important components of food. In later chapters, I'll explain how you can use specific neuronutrients as part of a broader plan to improve your mood and behavior.

It's important, however, that I emphasize that nutrition is not the only factor affecting your moods.

The way you eat has been shaped by your society, your family's eating habits, how stressed you are by work and your home life, and advertising. Basically, your eating habits did not develop in a vacuum. I refer to these cultural, psychological, and social influences as the *nutrisocial* factors that affect our eating habits. By understanding these nutrisocial factors—and some of them, like advertising, are very powerful—we can learn to ignore or resist them. I'll describe some of these nutrisocial forces in chapter 2 and offer advice for dealing with them in chapter 7.

What's Different about This Book

Over the last thirty years, numerous books have been written and published about food and mood. Most of these books have focused on using diets, vitamins, and herbs to treat depression. While depression is a common problem that can be addressed through safe alternative therapies, people suffer from many other mood and behavioral problems that make life difficult for them and the people in their lives. In *The Food-Mood Solution*, I tackle a variety of these more common mood problems, including

- Anger and hostile behavior
- Tension and anxiety
- Irritability and impatience
- Impulsive and distractible habits
- Fatigue and fuzzy thinking
- Stress and sleep problems
- Alcohol and drug abuse

This book is different from all the other food-mood books in another important way. In addition to providing practical nutrition advice to help improve your moods, I address many of the stresses that have set the stage for bad eating habits and, just as important, recommend specific ways for you to control the impact of these stresses on your life.

So, by the time you finish reading this book, how will you benefit? If you follow at least some of my advice, you will

- Deal more effectively with the inevitable stresses of life
- Have better and more stable moods
- Reduce your bad and down moods
- Be less irritable and impatient
- Gain more energy
- Sleep more soundly
- Be sharper mentally, with better concentration

Two-thirds of this book focuses on specific nutrition and lifestyle advice to help you think more clearly, have better moods, and develop the patience to treat other people fairly and reasonably, instead of taking your frustrations out on them. I recommend vitamins and other types of supplements, foods you should eat and those you should avoid, and lifestyle changes to help you slow down, unwind, and reprioritize. I firmly believe that my four-step program will foster both mental and physical health. It has worked for me and for many other people. I believe it will work for you.

Why I Wrote This Book

Although I originally trained to be a sociologist, with a strong emphasis on social and psychological behavior, I've spent more than thirty years writing about nutrition and health. I've long been fascinated by the interplay of society, behavior, eating habits, and health—including mental health. As I looked back at my own experiences, I realized that my moods and behavior were often close to the edge and occasionally erupted in anger.

As one example, when I was in my late forties, I was writing a book, going through a messy divorce, and dealing with a turbulent romantic relationship. I often felt overwhelmed by the stress in my life, and I was extremely anxious. I had to check my e-mail regularly—almost compulsively, for a reassuring or threatening message—and I always had my cell phone handy.

A turning point came one afternoon as I sat with a friend by a gentle stream in a desert canyon. At first, I was anxious about not being able to check my e-mail that morning, and adding to my initial distress, my cell phone LCD read "No service." But then I began to mellow. By the time I got home, I felt renewed as a human being. The experience reminded me how important it is to occasionally disconnect from the demands and pressures of life.

Meanwhile, as I looked at the world around me, I became dismayed by the increasing polarization in politics and religion. To me, these negative changes in the larger world reflect the increase in bad moods and behavior we experience in our personal encounters. The sociologist in me kicked in, and I started to think about how our national mood had deteriorated, along with our eating habits.

Over the years, I've been lucky to know and talk with many researchers and psychiatrists who have a keen understanding of how nutritional deficiencies or imbalances affect mood, perceptions, and behavior. I started to pay more attention to scientific and medical journal articles that explored the relationship between nutrition, biochemistry, mood, and behavior. At the same time, I was frustrated by advice in self-help and nutrition books that often discussed behavior or nutrition but not both. I saw that there was a need for a straightforward book that integrated practical nutrition and lifestyle tips to reduce stress and improve moods and behavior.

I can't blame all of the world's problems on bad eating habits. Our world has its share of political, economic, and religious strife, but we can certainly improve it in small ways that, with a little luck, will grow. These small acts start with us, with our eating habits and those of our families, and with learning how to achieve a personal sense of peace in a turbulent and moody world.

My message is really very simple: you can feel good. Armed with knowledge, you can succeed at anything.

PART I

The Food-Mood Connection

1

How Food Affects
Your Mood

Angie never had enough time to do everything she wanted to accomplish, and she always felt anxious and impatient. If she had to wait in line at the bank or the supermarket, she quickly got irritated and complained about the service. Angie routinely skipped meals and, when overly hungry, she drove through fast-food restaurants and practically inhaled her meals in the car. Then, after a few minutes, she usually felt so fuzzy and tired that she wanted to take a nap.

Jessica never felt right doing just one thing at a time. While driving, she also talked on her cell phone, sipped a soft drink, opened mail, or searched for a better song on her radio or CD player. Was she multitasking? No. She was addicted to impulsive behavior and couldn't focus on only one thing. It often got her into trouble. At work, her boss complained that she was always too distracted to complete tasks, and during the previous year, she had been in two fender benders because she wasn't paying attention to traffic.

Josh felt totally stressed by work. Every day he grabbed a cup of coffee on his way to the shop and later lived on candy bars, cans of soda pop, and burgers and fries. To try to keep up with his service calls, he drove too fast and regularly ran yellow and red lights, scaring and irking other drivers. At home, he was always irritable, and his wife and four-year-old daughter learned to give him plenty of space.

We've all known people like Angie, Jessica, and Josh (I'll come back to them later in the book). Their minds are in a jumble, and their moods and behavior disturb everyone around them. Sometimes we want to react to them, but most of the time we just want to get away as fast as possible.

If we look into the mirror, we just might admit that we have a little bit of Angie, Jessica, and Josh inside us, perhaps more than we would like. Sure, day-to-day stresses, a difficult boss, or an unhappy marriage can bring out the worst in anyone's behavior. But when life's daily activities bring out the dark sides of our personalities, it's time to think about changing before we hurt ourselves, our relationships, and the people around us.

Why do so many people have bad moods?

As I mentioned in the introduction, a big part of the reason is that eating bad—that is, unhealthful—foods often sets the stage for bad moods.

You're probably shaking your head and still wondering: how could food possibly affect mood?

Your brain is a biochemical thinking machine, and all of the biochemical building blocks of your brain eventually are affected by what you eat. Even the genes you inherited from your parents are influenced by what you put into your mouth. When you combine poor nutrition with stress—and who doesn't feel stressed these days?—normal brain activity, moods, and behavior get skewed. You probably know from experience that you're more likely to overreact to a situation when you're hungry than when you've just eaten.

How Blood Sugar Affects Your Mood

To make my point about how food affects mood, I often ask people how they feel after they eat and how they feel when they're hungry. Think about how your body and mind feel after you've eaten a meal or when you've skipped a meal. It may be very different from how you feel at other times.

Here are a couple of examples of how food affects mood.

After you eat lunch or dinner, odds are that you feel tired, your thinking becomes fuzzy, and your ability to concentrate decreases. Though common, these symptoms are not normal. So, what's happening? Your brain depends on a steady supply of blood sugar, or glucose, and the ideal amount of glucose falls within a fairly narrow range. When you eat too much food in one sitting or eat foods that contain too much sugar or sugarlike carbs—say, one slice of pizza too many—your blood sugar rises too high. When that happens, your brain fuzzes out, you get drowsy, and you naturally want to take a nap. It's a little like having your body and brain circuits overloaded with too many sugars.

The opposite—low blood sugar—isn't good, either. When glucose falls below the normal range, you get hungry. Then, if you don't eat within a reasonable amount of time, your glucose drops even lower. Without enough fuel for your brain, your mental activity actually shifts to a more primitive and less sociable level. You're likely to become impatient, irritable, and aggressive and may react to other people in anger. You might also feel physically tired, shaky, and weak. In ancient times, low blood sugar was a sign that it was time to hunt or gather food. Today, low glucose is particularly bad if you're stressed out and can't eat for a while, such as when you're stuck in traffic during the late-afternoon rush hour.

Your blood sugar normally fluctuates a little during the course of a day. But when you eat the wrong kinds of foods—particularly foods high in sugars and sugarlike carbs—your blood sugar swings can be extreme and frequent. People who experience these blood sugar swings sense when they're feeling a little weak or when their mood is about to go south, and, out of habit, they often reach for a soft drink or a candy bar to quickly raise their glucose. But candy bars and energy bars are only temporary fixes, and they actually make blood sugar swings even worse.

Whenever you have bad or down moods, they can affect your outward behavior. An angry comment or outburst can cause hurt feelings, start an argument, or even trigger a physical brawl. Often, the effect snowballs.

You know how frustrating it is when someone cuts you off in traffic or doesn't let you easily merge onto the freeway. When people are mean to you, you may want to vent your anger at the nearest innocent driver.

It's no coincidence that we see so many bad moods during the morning and the afternoon commute. Traffic congestion is stressful. In the morning, that stress may be compounded by a breakfast of coffee and sugary foods, leading to blood sugar swings. In the afternoon, people are again tired and hungry, and their neuronutrient levels are declining.

> ### Quick Tip
> **A Better Fix for Blood Sugar Swings**
> Instead of a soft drink or a sugary snack, eat some unsalted mixed nuts or a slice of deli turkey and cheese. These foods help to stabilize blood sugar. It's also good to start your day with protein, such as eggs or a couple of slices of deli turkey.

Take the Mood Quiz

This five-part quiz will help you assess your moods and some of the dietary and nondietary factors that affect your moods and behavior. Circle either "Y" for yes or "N" for no. Answer the questions honestly, and use a separate piece of paper if you don't want other people to see your answers.

How Stressed Are You?

I feel like I have too much to do at work.	Y/N
I feel like I have too much to do at home.	Y/N
I feel like people ask me to do too many things.	Y/N
I often wonder how I'm going to get everything done.	Y/N
When I'm driving, I often get impatient with and annoyed by slow drivers.	Y/N
When I'm in a hurry, I often run yellow and red lights.	Y/N
Sometimes I do things that scare the hell out of me.	Y/N
I often use my cell phone while driving.	Y/N

I've gotten at least one speeding ticket or caused a car
     accident in the past year.   Y/N

I really get annoyed with people who are slow in line.   Y/N

I don't have the time to do everything I need to do.   Y/N

Sometimes I just want to scream in frustration.   Y/N

There are times when I realize I'm jumpy and jittery.   Y/N

I don't get as much sleep as I should.   Y/N

Some of my relationships, such as with my spouse, friends,
     and coworkers, are not as good as they used to be.   Y/N

Explanation: A certain degree of stress in today's world is normal. If you circled yes for any of these questions, you're under some stress. If you've circled yes to more than a few of the questions, you're under a lot of stress! Constant stress takes a toll on your neurotransmitters, neuronutrients, eating habits, and physical health. As you read this book, incorporate my recommendations for reducing or buffering your stresses.

What Are Your Moods Like?

People have said that I'm moody.   Y/N

People have said that I have difficulty in relationships.   Y/N

I feel tense or anxious a lot of the time.   Y/N

I often feel down or depressed.   Y/N

I hate doing nothing because I tend to get bored and fidget.   Y/N

I usually respond immediately to e-mails or text messages.   Y/N

I always answer my cell phone, regardless of where I am.   Y/N

I get irritated by people who are slow.   Y/N

A lot of people rub me the wrong way.   Y/N

I get annoyed, pissed off, or angry at least once a week.   Y/N

I like destroying things or watching things get destroyed
     or wrecked.   Y/N

I've unintentionally scared the hell out of other people.   Y/N

I drink more than normal amounts of alcohol or use illegal
    drugs at least once a day.   Y/N

Explanation: We all have our moments because life can be trying. If
you circled yes for at least two of these questions, though, it's a sign that
you're often in a bad mood or you have frequent mood swings. As you
read this book, pay special attention to the supplements and the eating
habits that can improve your moods. They will make you more fun to
live with—and will make it easier for you to live with yourself.

What Are Your Eating Habits Like?

I usually skip breakfast or just have some coffee.   Y/N

I like convenience foods because I don't have time to eat
    a regular meal.   Y/N

My usual breakfast includes a breakfast bar, an energy bar,
    cereal, or something sweet.   Y/N

I eat at fast-food restaurants (e.g., McDonald's or Burger
    King) at least twice a week.   Y/N

A lot of the foods I eat at home come in a box, a bottle,
    or a jar.   Y/N

I drink sugary (nondiet) soft drinks on a regular basis.   Y/N

I drink more than two cups of coffee on most days.   Y/N

I like eating fries.   Y/N

I really enjoy and eat a lot of bread, pasta, or pizza.   Y/N

I usually crave something sweet between meals or often
    have other types of food cravings.   Y/N

I usually eat my meals quickly and don't linger over them.   Y/N

I tend to feel tired after eating.   Y/N

Explanation: These questions provide clues to your overall eating
habits. If you've answered yes to any of them, your eating habits are not
as healthy as they could be. Many of these eating habits set you up for a
diabetes-like blood sugar pattern, which can increase fuzzy thinking and
mood swings.

What's the Rest of Your Life Like?

I don't have enough time to unwind.	Y/N
I think about work on my days off and when I'm on vacation.	Y/N
I feel like I need to check work-related e-mail or voice mail on weekends or when I'm on vacation.	Y/N
I don't exercise regularly.	Y/N
I don't have many hobbies, and I don't do much aside from work other than maybe watch sports on television or go out drinking with friends.	Y/N
It has been a while since I've had a good hearty laugh with my friends or significant other.	Y/N
I don't have any close friends I can really open up with and talk about how I feel inside.	Y/N

Explanation: Answering yes to at least one of these questions suggests that you may be too preoccupied with work or your life isn't balanced enough to offset stresses. When you don't have a variety of interesting activities in your life, you are more likely to have mood and physical problems related to too much stress. If you've answered yes to two or more questions, your overall lifestyle may set the stage for mood and behavior problems.

How Do You Feel Physically?

I usually have trouble getting up in the morning.	Y/N
I often have headaches, heartburn, or an upset stomach.	Y/N
I am overweight and at least some of the weight is around my belly.	Y/N
I take at least one prescription medicine each day for a chronic health problem.	Y/N
I've been diagnosed with high cholesterol, triglycerides, or blood pressure.	Y/N
I don't have a lot of energy, and I often feel like I have to push myself to get things done.	Y/N

I am usually very tired by the time I get to bed.   Y/N

I keep waking up and have trouble getting a good night's
sleep.   Y/N

Explanation: Answering yes to two or more of these questions suggests that your eating habits are not ideal and may be pushing you toward a diabetes-like blood sugar pattern. Elevated blood fats and blood pressure, as well as a lack of energy, are often signs of blood sugar problems. Even if your mood is relatively stable now, you may eventually develop mood problems.

The Bigger Picture

I don't mean to suggest that nutrition is the only factor influencing our moods. To the contrary, our eating habits and other types of behavior result from a complex interplay of nutrition, genetics, upbringing, psychological makeup, stresses, society, and the people around us.

Stresses at work or at home burn up (through increased chemical reactions) many mood-calming neurotransmitters and neuronutrients at a faster-than-normal rate. Furthermore, when we feel stressed, good eating habits are usually the first thing we sacrifice. That's because stress distracts us from eating healthy foods and eating at regular times. We'll hold off on lunch or even skip it. The irony is that when we need more neuronutrients to buffer stress, we actually end up consuming less.

It's also important to understand that our moods are affected by many other nutritional factors besides blood sugar levels. Virtually every vitamin and mineral has an impact on our brain function, but some nutrients have particularly powerful effects. Low levels of these important neuronutrients reduce the brain's production of mood-enhancing neurotransmitters.

Nutrition, Health, and Mood

One difficulty in the field of nutrition is that many consequences of poor eating habits take years to appear. People won't get fat or have a heart attack after eating just one fast-food meal, so they (doctors included)

don't always see a clear cause-and-effect relationship between unhealthy foods and illness.

It's a different story, though, when it comes to nutrition and mood. That's because *the first signs of nutritional deficiencies and imbalances are usually altered moods and behavior*. Yet we rarely pay attention to how food affects our moods and thinking.

This connection between nutrition and mood has been demonstrated by many scientists, including the late Nobel laureate Linus Pauling, Ph.D., and David Benton, Ph.D., a psychology professor at the University of Wales, Swansea. Benton conducted a variety of experiments on his students, who seemed to be in generally good physical and mental health. He found that their moods improved substantially after they began taking a daily high-potency multivitamin supplement.

Other researchers, including William Walsh, Ph.D., of the Pfeiffer Treatment Center in Warrenville, Illinois, and Bernard Gesch, Ph.D., of Oxford University, England, have consistently found that vitamin supplements can even reduce aggressive and violent criminal behavior. If vitamins and good eating habits can improve the most serious mood and behavior problems, imagine how they could help you cope with

The Fast-Food Junk-Food Cascade

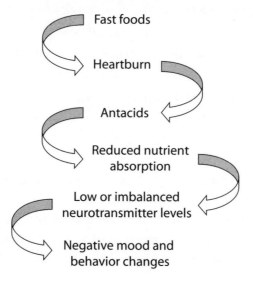

Fast foods

Heartburn

Antacids

Reduced nutrient absorption

Low or imbalanced neurotransmitter levels

Negative mood and behavior changes

run-of-the-mill stresses of modern life, such as a hectic schedule, traffic jams, and Machiavellian office politics.

I'll describe more of this fascinating research in later chapters. The point I want to make, however, is that merely taking a high-potency multivitamin supplement can greatly improve the moods of many—perhaps most—people.

Which Types of Mood Problems May Be Food-Related?

Many mood and behavioral problems are actually connected to each other. Sometimes the differences are only in degree, such as the progression from irritability to anger. I've organized some of the most common mood and behavioral issues into related groups.

- *Anger disorders* include irritability, crankiness, resentment, brooding, rudeness, aggressiveness, road rage, juvenile delinquency, and criminal violence.

- *Impulsive and distractible disorders* include rash behavior, some types of irrational behavior, excessive multitasking, some types of addiction, and adult attention-deficit hyperactivity disorder (ADHD).

- *Anxiety disorders* include tension, jumpiness, worry, fear, panic attacks, post-traumatic stress disorders, and obsessive-compulsive behavior (such as repeated and unnecessary checking).

- *Depression-related disorders* include down days, various intensities of depression, and bipolar (manic-depressive) disorder.

- *Fatigue, tiredness, and mental fuzziness* include regular feelings of tiredness and mental fatigue, difficulty concentrating (especially after eating), poor memory, feeling spacey, and overeating.

The Canary in the Mine . . . and in the Mind

Recognizing that you or someone close to you regularly has bad moods is a lot like paying attention to the "canary in the mine." Years ago, miners took canaries deep into mines because the birds were particularly sensitive to poison gas. If a canary died, it was a warning for the miners to immediately evacuate.

Many doctors understand that certain mood or personality traits are strongly associated with a person's physical health. For example, people who are depressed are more likely than nondepressed individuals to develop heart disease or cancer, and quick-tempered men are more likely than others to drop dead from sudden heart attacks. Yet the relationship between mood and physical illness is far more intriguing and interesting.

Unhealthy changes in mood and behavior are often the canary in the mind. The nutritional deficiencies and imbalances that produce mood and behavior problems sow the seeds for physical diseases, such as heart disease and cancer, years later. This shouldn't be all that surprising because the same nutrient-rich or nutrient-weak blood that flows through the brain also flows through the rest of the body. The difference is that the brain is very sensitive to poor nutrition, whereas it takes years for poor nutrition to affect the heart and other organs.

Nutritional Deficiencies Are Common

I've suggested that large numbers of people are poorly nourished, and you may wonder whether the situation is really that bad. After all, we've often been told that our country is the best-fed nation in the world.

Unfortunately, the situation is far worse than most people realize. Part of the reason is our growing consumption of fast foods, convenience foods, soft drinks, and other junk foods, which are typically high in sugars and sugarlike carbs and low in protein, fiber, and vitamins. At the very least, junk foods displace healthier and more nutritious foods that contain lots of neuronutrients; however, junk foods also interfere with how the body uses essential nutrients.

We've been told that nutritional deficiencies are prevalent in developing and poor nations, and we believe that they are rare in modern Western nations. The truth is that nutritional deficiencies and imbalances are relatively common in the United States, and they set the stage for a variety of physical and psychological problems. Although Canadians and Western Europeans are, as a whole, healthier than Americans, they increasingly suffer the same fate of modern malnutrition. The cause, in large part, is related to the worldwide distribution and consumption of

American junk foods, from soft drinks to burgers and fries. Such convenience foods displace more nutritious foods.

In the United States, three-fourths of Americans do not consume the extremely minute yet required daily amount of folic acid, a key B vitamin that is involved in maintaining good moods. Similarly, almost half of us don't get enough vitamin C, about one-third don't consume enough vitamin B6, and almost a third don't have enough vitamin B12 in their diets. All of these vitamins are essential neuronutrients.

The graph below, compiled from data on a U.S. Department of Agriculture Web site, reflects the percentages of people who do *not* consume the minimum amounts of vitamins and minerals recommended by the government. Because the government's standards are cautious and conservative, however, there's good reason to believe that the percentages of people with deficiencies are even higher.

Still other factors take a toll on our neuronutrients. Most over-the-counter and prescription drugs either reduce the absorption of nutrients or interfere with how the body uses them, thus increasing the likelihood of multiple vitamin and mineral deficiencies. Some of these drugs are taken routinely by millions of people. Antacids and related drugs (such as Prilosec) for the treatment of heartburn and gastric reflux impede the absorption of vitamin C and the B vitamins. So do oral antibiotics, and

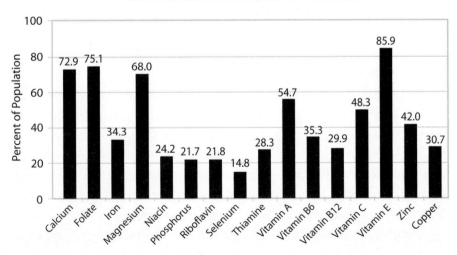

Percentage of Americans Not Consuming the Recommended Intakes of Nutrients

their effects on B-vitamin absorption can last months and years after a two-week regimen. Oral contraceptives, analgesics, and cholesterol-lowering drugs also hinder a variety of normal biochemical processes that impact both the brain and the body. All of these drugs further compromise our neuronutrients. Side effects are often a result of how certain drugs prevent nutrients from working normally.

Nutrition, Brain Nutrients, and Moods

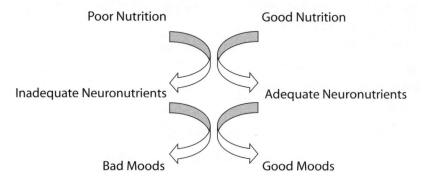

Poor Nutrition   Good Nutrition

Inadequate Neuronutrients   Adequate Neuronutrients

Bad Moods   Good Moods

When you add the neuronutrient-robbing effect of our day-to-day stresses, it's easy to believe that millions of people are literally running on fumes, nutritionally speaking. For a variety of reasons, such as genetics or upbringing, a few people are more likely than others to be the canaries—more prone to having road rage, being involved in high-speed car chases, "going postal," and committing other irrational and senseless acts. Worse, as more people suffer from deteriorating nutritional health, still greater numbers of people are negatively affected—hence, the increase in bad moods.

The situation may sound grim, but most of this book focuses on what you, as an individual, can do to change it.

Our Amazing Neurotransmitters

Our moods, thoughts, and memories are ultimately based on the chemistry of the brain. This isn't meant to belittle the importance of your feelings, your thoughts, or your uniqueness as a human being. Your feelings are as real as the book you're holding, your computer, or your car. My point is simply that the workings of your brain are the result of chemical reactions shaped by your diet, your genetics, and your experiences. For example, your experiences influence your brain chemistry, and your brain chemistry affects your moods and reactions.

Everything we experience modifies the brain's chemistry, recording an impression and usually prompting a reaction. If you're in love, brain chemicals create a sense of euphoria similar to a drug-induced high. In contrast, the rapid heartbeat and fear you experience when you see flashing police lights results from a near-instant rush of adrenaline, a powerful hormone and neurotransmitter.

Remember, all of our neurotransmitters are influenced by what we eat. They depend on vitamins, minerals, protein, healthy fats, and a small amount of high-quality carbohydrates.

How Are Men and Women Different in Their Moods and Behavior?

Men and women have obvious biological differences. Our moods and behavior are hardwired by our biology and genetics, and are soft-wired

How Angie Learned to Settle Down

Angie, whom you read about at the beginning of this chapter, was always anxious and impatient. She regularly skipped meals and ended up driving through fast-food restaurants to eat just as her blood sugar was crashing. Then she usually felt fuzzy brained and wanted to take a nap.

She eventually sought the advice of a nutritionally oriented physician for her bouts of fatigue. He and his nutritionist recommended better meal planning, more protein and fresh vegetables, and supplements containing B vitamins, magnesium, and L-theanine.

Her response to eating more protein—a rotisserie chicken and steamed vegetables on the first day—was nothing short of dramatic. She slept more soundly and woke up feeling alert and energetic. By eating two scrambled eggs for breakfast, she was able to sustain her mental clarity and energy through early afternoon. Several months later, Angie's sister described her as a new person.

by our upbringing and socialization. The result is a mix of patterns attributed to our sex and individual traits. Following are some common differences between men's and women's moods and behavior. Please understand that these general patterns do not universally apply to all men or women.

- Men are more likely than women to express anger through physically aggressive behavior. Women get angry, but they are more likely to express it as sarcasm or passive-aggressive behavior.

- Women are more likely to express sadness and depression because it is socially acceptable for women to talk about their feelings. Men have difficulty expressing sadness and depression because they were usually raised without learning how to express their emotions.

- Men are more likely than women to feel depressed because of anxieties, such as worries about work, relationships, sexual performance, and appearance.

- Women are more likely to deal with depression by overeating. Men are more likely to deal with depression by drinking alcohol.

- Men are more likely to become withdrawn when wrestling with anxiety or depression. They are less likely than women to talk about their emotions and to seek professional help.

- Women are more likely to seek professional help, such as psychological counseling. Men have a higher rate of suicide, partly because they internalize (rather than express) their feelings.

- Men are less likely than women to be aware of their relationship-dependency needs.

- Women's moods are more likely to be influenced by some aspects of their biology, such as menstrual periods, pregnancy, postpregnancy, and menopause.

The many stresses in our lives lead to neuronutrient and neurotransmitter imbalances, which set the stage for chronic mood problems. But how many of us really think about the price we pay for all this stress? The next chapter looks at some of these stresses and how they blind us to their health consequences.

2

How Life's Stresses Do a Number on Your Moods

Good nutrition may underpin normal brain chemistry, moods, and behavior, but our eating habits don't exist in a vacuum. Rather, they are shaped by many nutrisocial factors, including upbringing, education, peer pressure, food advertising, and how much (or how little) time we have to cook and eat. We may not be able to alter these nutrisocial forces; however, once we are aware of them, we can limit their impact on us and on our family members.

The Nutrisocial Roots of Mood and Behavior Problems

The bad moods and behavior that are rampant today result largely from a collision between the stress of contemporary life and nutritional deficiencies and imbalances, which reduce our resistance to this stress. Many of our day-to-day decisions and activities are driven by anxiety, worry, fear, and boredom, all of which alter our eating habits and place greater demands on our nutrient-dependent neurotransmitters. As our calming neuronutrients get used up, we become less likely to act reasonable and more likely to revert to primitive and aggressive behavior. Studies have confirmed that when we're stressed, we tend to lose self-control.

Changes throughout History in the Foods We Eat

Ever since the Romans perfected the refining of grains two thousand years ago, foods have been increasingly processed through mechanical and chemical means. Such processing and refining reduce the amount of neuronutrients in foods and increase the amount of rapidly digested sugars and carbohydrates—changes that play havoc with our blood sugar levels and our moods.

What do I mean by processing and refining? An apple is an unrefined food. When it's made into applesauce, much of the fiber is broken down, so our bodies absorb the sugars faster in a way that's more likely to cause a diabetic-like glucose spike. During the processing of applesauce, levels of vitamin C and other nutrients decrease. Further refining removes all fiber, resulting in sugary apple juice that is little different from a soft drink. As another example, wheat grains are impossible for us to chew—our teeth weren't designed for breaking them down. Mechanical processing and refining removes the most nutritious part of the grain, as does bleaching to turn brownish flour white. The resulting white flour and bread have few nutrients and contain a type of starch that's absorbed similarly to pure sugar.

The processing of foods accelerated about a hundred years ago with the invention of new industrial equipment and techniques, and food processing has only increased over the last sixty years. The first true convenience meal, a TV dinner, was marketed in the 1950s, about the same time that McDonald's fast-food restaurants began to dot the landscape. For many years, the negative health effects of nutritionally altered foods were offset by a decline in cigarette smoking; however, the preponderance of unhealthful foods has since led to epidemics of obesity and diabetes—which contribute to bad moods.

Changes in the Way We Live

Significant social changes, beginning in the 1970s, paralleled and encouraged changes in our eating habits. Consumer expectations rose (such as for bigger houses, newer cars, and larger televisions), which led to greater numbers of dual-career couples. After all, two people could make more money and achieve a higher standard of living compared with one worker and a stay-at-home spouse. Yet dual-career families often experience more stress because, in addition to both partners working, they must also juggle parenthood, shopping, cooking, laundry, and other chores.

By the early 1990s, when domestic and global business climates became especially cutthroat, the pace of business increased sharply, leading to shorter turnaround times. Companies demanded more productivity and time from their employees in order to remain competitive. In the process, everything in our lives sped up—we segued from telephone calls and regular mail to the routine use of overnight deliveries and faxes, and now to cell phones, e-mails, and instant messages. Service companies routinely promise 24/7 service, and many employees remain in touch with their companies and customers on evenings and weekends. All of this adds stress and takes a toll on our neuronutrients and neurotransmitters.

In 1970, in his prescient book *Future Shock*, Alvin Toffler observed that the increasing speed of social change feels overwhelming. He wrote that it can lead to confusion, disorientation, and distorted perceptions of reality, all characterized by symptoms of fatigue, anxiety, tenseness, or extreme irritability. Toffler was predicting the world we now live in.

Nutrisocial Pressure Points

When we feel stressed, we invariably sacrifice our eating habits, sometimes by making less healthful food choices and other times by skipping or delaying meals. When we're faced with too many tasks at home and at work, we usually reduce the time needed to plan and prepare meals and instead opt for convenience and fast foods. When we spend less time cooking, we're also less likely to teach our children how to cook or appreciate fresh foods. In this way, the impact of today's pressures will affect subsequent generations.

One hundred years ago, people cooked nearly all their meals at home from scratch. Our dependence on prepared foods has increased significantly, and from the 1980s through the present, the consumption of fast foods (e.g., McDonald's and Burger King) and convenience foods (e.g., microwave meals, breakfast bars) has grown at an astonishing rate, supplanting home-cooked meals. Only about one-third of all dinners are now completely homemade, and 7 percent of these meals are nothing more than sandwiches. One-fourth of home meals are actually purchased frozen or prepared at a restaurant or a market, and the number of take-out meals from restaurants has increased by two-thirds over the last twenty years. We suffer serious neuronutritional consequences because of our poor eating habits.

The Starbucks Syndrome

As people did their best to navigate the mounting demands of work and home life, they sacrificed many aspects of a balanced life. The average American now sleeps about ninety minutes less each night than the typical person did in 1900. The National Sleep Foundation has reported that three-fourths of young and middle-aged women get less than eight hours of sleep each night and, not surprisingly, feel tired all the time.

Being tired is comparable to being drunk—it affects our thinking, reflexes, and behavior. Studies have shown that a person who is tired and drives a car has reflexes comparable to someone who has had too much to drink. People often combat this fatigue the way drunks do—by drinking coffee and soft drinks (many of which combine caffeine and sugars) to temporarily boost energy levels and improve mental sharpness. Caffeine also increases the secretion of adrenaline and cortisol, while decreasing levels of calming neurotransmitters, such as serotonin and GABA. Tired, stimulated, and distracted, the mind becomes a jumble.

Just about everyone knows that too much caffeine has side effects, including headaches and an edgy feeling. While doctors don't seem particularly interested in diagnosing coffee addiction or "Starbucks syndrome," some psychiatrists have argued that caffeine withdrawal should be listed as an official psychiatric diagnosis. They have pointed out that various symptoms, such as irritability, depression, muscle pain, migraines and other types of headaches, and even flulike symptoms, can be triggered when people miss their caffeine fix.

The increasing consumption of caffeine led to yet another problem: not only were people sleeping less, but they were also sleeping less restfully. Sugary foods and irregular and late-evening meals compounded the problem, exacerbating morning hypoglycemia (low blood sugar) and hyperglycemia (elevated blood sugar) and making it more difficult to get out of bed. For many people, the only solution was to start another day with coffee.

Marketing through Anxiety

Still other factors have contributed to our feelings of stress. In recent years, people have developed an unusually high level of general anxiety—a vague sense of nervousness, jumpiness, and fear—which places further demands on our neurotransmitters. This anxiety goes beyond how the threat of crime or terrorism has affected our lives.

This background anxiety has to a great extent been fostered by two factors: the increased use of fear to sell various products, and the clever use of fear and uncertainty on television and radio. Fear is one of the most primal and powerful of all emotions, and it triggers the release of stress hormones, which affect everything from mood to heart rate. Tapping into or creating fear in order to market products has become one of the most common advertising techniques, and the resulting anxiety now permeates our lives.

The Increase in Fear, Uncertainty, and Doubt

The use of anxiety to sell products goes back about thirty years. Until that time, companies generally promoted the benefits of their products, such as better cars, bigger television screens, and more stylish clothing. In the 1970s, IBM developed a marketing concept known as FUD. The acronym might sound funny, but it stands for fear, uncertainty, and doubt. This marketing strategy aroused fears, uncertainties, and doubts about buying non-IBM products. The whole point of FUD was to convince customers that bad things would happen if they didn't buy IBM products. Using FUD to sell products was very shrewd. Instead of emphasizing the merits of a product, FUD tapped into customers' fears about making the wrong purchase decision.

The FUD concept succeeded so well that it is now used to sell almost every imaginable product, from tooth whiteners to paper shredders to prescription drugs. Even iPods use the fear of not looking cool as a marketing technique. Talk radio, argumentative cable news shows, and news teasers all use FUD to sell products and to keep people tuned in. If you're told there's an upcoming story affecting your health or finances, or a breaking crime story, you will probably be worried enough to listen.

It might seem easy enough to ignore advertising, television, and radio, but FUD has found a susceptible audience in millions of Americans. Our excessive consumption of caffeine and sugary foods, combined with a low intake of neuronutrients, lays the groundwork for feeling jumpy. When we're primed for anxiety, it doesn't take much to exploit that anxiety and turn us into a nation of nervous wrecks.

A Sense of Overwhelming Stress

All of the foregoing factors help to make us overly susceptible to individual sources of stress, but what exactly makes something stressful?

Stress is often the social and psychological pressure to do things we really don't want to do, as well as to do too much in an unreasonably short amount of time. Some stress is inevitable because life requires compromise, and other types of stress (such as my deadline in writing this book) actually push us to greater creativity and accomplishments. For most of us, however, stress pushes us out of a zone in which we feel calm, relaxed, satisfied, and happy, and it takes a toll on our physical health and emotional well-being.

Stress places a greater demand on our calming neurotransmitters, burning them up (along with their nutritional building blocks) faster than when we are not stressed. *As our calming neurotransmitters decline, our stimulating ones dominate by default, creating an imbalance that can alter how we think, feel, and act.* The negative effect can continue long after the stressful experience, such as when we stay resentful or angry.

Biologically, we favor stimulating neurotransmitters, and caffeine, sugar, and stress arouse us. In ancient times, being anxious and aggressive helped sharpen and protect us against predators or other attackers, and therefore these traits were related to survival. If we were depressed, we'd be too sluggish to respond.

Many people turn to alcohol, drugs, or cigarettes to ease their stress, but in the long run these substances exacerbate the damage. Sometimes people become addicted to the adrenaline high that can accompany stress, and restless people might seek out stressful situations or generate internal feelings of stress when there is no outside stress.

Although most stresses have an external source, such as work, we can usually control our responses to them. Stress does not have to dominate our lives, and we can improve our resistance to it by modifying our diet and lifestyle.

Quick Tip

The Serenity Prayer
You've probably heard the Serenity Prayer, written in 1932 by Reinhold Niebuhr: "God, grant me the serenity to accept the things I cannot change, the courage to change the things I can, and the wisdom to know the difference."

This prayer is actually advice for how to deal with conflict and stress, so that we make sound decisions about what we are capable of changing (to reduce stress) and what we must learn to accept (also to reduce stress).

What Happens When We're Stressed?

In the animal kingdom, psychological and emotional stresses are usually fleeting. When a lion chases a deer, the deer immediately releases large amounts of stress hormones, including adrenaline. These chemicals heighten the animal's physical fight-or-flight response and also function as neurotransmitters that sharpen decision making, such as figuring out how to escape. If the deer successfully gets away, its stress hormones quickly decline, and the animal calms down and resumes grazing.

Like animals, we are biologically designed to use these powerful chemicals in short bursts to counter stress and ensure survival. In our modern world, however, we deal with stress at every turn: at home, while commuting, at work, when looking for a parking space, while shopping, while waiting in line, and even when we grab a quick bite to eat. It often seems as if most people feel stressed nearly every moment of their waking lives. Under chronic stress, the body secretes stress hormones almost all the time.

When we secrete high levels of stress hormones for weeks, months, or years, they stop protecting us and instead start to damage the body. Elevated levels of the stress hormone cortisol are particularly toxic to brain cells. Cortisol interferes with the production of new brain cells, shrinks brain size, and hinders thinking and memory. Chronic stress makes us more anxious, jumpy, fearful, and impatient—and later, fuzzy and fatigued.

Elevated cortisol levels have other undesirable effects as well. Cortisol activity is intertwined with insulin, and cortisol increases both blood sugar and insulin levels, eventually leading to more belly fat and a greater risk of diabetes. Belly fat is a telltale sign of abnormal fluctuations of blood sugar and insulin levels, prediabetes, and full-blown type-2 diabetes, all of which can negatively affect thinking processes, concentration, mood, behavior, and energy levels. Chronically high levels of cortisol also lower levels of DHEA (dehydroepiandrosterone), a hormone that helps us to maintain youthfulness and sexuality and resist stress, and protects us against depression.

Are You Stressed?

For many people, that's an easy question to answer. If you feel like you're stressed, you probably are. If you're not sure, ask yourself whether you are often tense, rush to get things done, have too many things to do, or feel tired most of the time. If this sounds like you, you're stressed.

According to surveys, three-fourths of Americans describe their work as stressful, and one-fourth of employees believe that work is their main source of stress. Up to 90 percent of visits to primary care physicians are for health problems related to stress. In England, 58 percent of workers complain about work-related stress.

Why the emphasis on stress? In a manner of speaking, stress is the hammer that drives the nail, and the nail is what makes us want to scream. Is it any wonder that, at the end of a stressful day, some people describe themselves as "feeling hammered?" They feel beaten up and in pain.

As people feel more stressed, they lose self-control. Researchers have confirmed that stressed people are more likely to go off their diets, drink more coffee, smoke more cigarettes, ignore household chores, neglect commitments with friends, and become financially irresponsible. They also tend to be moody, irritable, angry, and aggressive. Stress destroys stable moods and emotional equilibrium.

Multitasking as Irrational, Stress-Promoting Behavior

By the 1980s, businesses were encouraging their employees to multi-task—that is, to do more than one task at a time—and the pressure to multitask has since gotten worse. A typical multitasker might be writing an e-mail, talking on the phone, and eating lunch at his desk. Multitasking was seen by management as a way to increase productivity, and on the surface, it certainly seemed to do that. It has become part of the culture of countless corporations. Yet studies have consistently found that multitasking actually decreases productivity, whereas completing tasks serially (one at a time) allows you to get more done in the same amount of time.

By promoting and rewarding multitasking, businesses encouraged behavior that had striking similarities to certain aspects of adult ADHD (attention-deficit hyperactivity disorder). While it's relatively easy to get people to adopt what is essentially impulsive and distractible behavior, it's extremely difficult to break these habits. Furthermore, diets that are low in neuronutrients help to maintain the anxiety that drives this ADHD-like behavior.

The habit of multitasking migrated from work to other parts of our lives, and now many people don't feel right unless they always do more than one thing at a time, such as talk on a cell phone, eat, or apply makeup while driving to work. If you've driven behind someone who is multitasking, though, you know that the driver is not paying attention to traffic conditions. Multitaskers cannot give any single task their full attention, and it shows in their reduced performance. That's why multitasking is less efficient.

Multitasking has morphed into yet another behavior, one that is best described as impulsive/addictive and that also resembles aspects of ADHD. For example, many people are so addicted to e-mail that they constantly interrupt their work or other activities to impulsively check e-mails (that is, to give themselves distractions) or to read and send instant messages. Similarly, many people are addicted to their cell phones and always have to be talking with someone or must answer (be distracted by) every call, regardless of what they are doing at the time. Often, people feel anxious and jittery when they aren't multitasking, and this anxiety bears a strong similarity to being addicted to tobacco, alcohol, or another drug and needing a hit. I'll return to this subject in chapter 13.

Other Common Stresses

We face many other common stresses in our lives. Following are several more, and I'm sure you can create your own list of stressful situations.

- *Stress at work.* For years, people have called these work pressures a rat race, but the situation has hit a new and ignominious low with 24/7. Rather than being a badge of honor, 24/7 is really a sign of how perverted and stressful the workplace has become. To successfully compete, many companies cannot afford to sleep (after all, the rest of the world is awake and working), and fewer workers can afford to be out of touch on weekends or vacation.

  Newspaper and magazine headlines have conveyed the pervasiveness of the problem with such headlines as "Eight Isn't Enough in Today's Jobs," "Ground Down by Daily Grind," and "Is There Life after Work?" Further contributing to the problem are the stresses of office politics and bullying bosses, which have been described in newspaper articles in the United States, England, and Ireland.

- *Stress in personal relationships.* Difficulties in interpersonal relationships are another common source of stress that literally drains us of neuronutrients. Some conflicts are inevitable when any two people, with their inevitable differences, interact in very personal and intimate ways. In healthy relationships, the occasional disagreement is usually resolved or forgotten; however, regular arguments and resentments add to feelings of stress. Many relationship conflicts boil down to a couple of fundamental issues, such as poor communication and trying to control the other person.

- *Stress from a lack of rest.* Stress and elevated cortisol levels disrupt sleep, and a lack of sleep further raises cortisol levels. It's a vicious cycle. Both cortisol and inadequate sleep are associated with a greater likelihood of developing obesity, diabetes, and heart disease.

  Taking a vacation is the traditional valve that lets us release the accumulated stresses of work, but work pressures and anxieties actually keep many people from taking vacations. According to a survey by Oxford Health Plans, 20 percent of Americans have too much work to do and don't use all of the vacation time they've earned. Many people don't want to take time off because they dread the work that will be waiting for them when they return. Others simply don't take vacations, or if they do, they take their laptop, cell phone, and BlackBerry with them.

- *Stress from commuting.* Commuting to and from work, particularly in cars, is another regular stress for millions of people. It's frustrating to be stuck in traffic and powerless to do anything about it (especially when our blood sugar is low before dinner), and this stress takes a toll on our neuronutrients and neurotransmitters.

  A survey conducted in 2005 found that the typical Los Angeles car commuter spends almost a hundred hours each year stuck in traffic jams. I once had a job with an eighty-mile round-trip commute. On the best days, the commute took only one hour each way. After eight years, I realized that I was spending one-seventh of my life in a car, and I began to look for another job.

Why Comfort Foods Are Appealing

When we feel stressed, we are more likely to seek out comfort foods—specifically those high in sugars, carbohydrates, and fats—as an antidote.

Comfort foods temporarily reduce feelings of stress, which is no doubt why we find them so comforting. Some research suggests that eating comfort foods is comparable to self-medicating our stress wounds. Yet there is a serious downside: the regular consumption of comfort foods leads to unstable blood sugar and insulin levels and can contribute to overweight and mood swings.

The combination of high cortisol and insulin levels causes sugar to be stored as fat in the belly, instead of on the hips or the buttocks. Belly fat, a sign of Syndrome X (sometimes called metabolic syndrome or insulin-resistance syndrome), elevates cholesterol and triglycerides and increases the risk of diabetes and heart disease. (See my book *Syndrome X: The Complete Nutritional Program to Prevent and Reverse Insulin Resistance.*) Because Syndrome X is a form of prediabetes, it frequently includes mood changes, such as impatience, irritability, anger, hostility, and fuzzy thinking.

The ideal solution is not to self-medicate with foods that promote mood swings or heart disease, but rather to reduce or eliminate the source of stress, a topic that I'll address later in this book.

In the next chapter, I will explain more about neurotransmitters and will describe some of the nutrients needed to make them. Under ideal circumstances, neurotransmitters exist in balance with one another, shifting somewhat to help us adapt to life's changing situations. Problems arise when certain neurotransmitters remain at very high or low levels, leading to inappropriate moods and behavior.

3

Neuronutrients, Moods, and Your Mind

Psychiatrists often prescribe medications to alter neurotransmitter levels in the brain and to improve mood and behavior. Yet it is actually much more straightforward, effective, and safe to use neuronutrients—the nutritional building blocks of neurotransmitters.

Neurotransmitters are some of the most amazing natural biochemicals in our bodies. These chemical messengers are used by brain and nerve cells to communicate with one another. Neurotransmitters convey information about our environment. They tell us when we touch something hot or sharp or whether we should feel safe or in danger. Released by one cell, neurotransmitters attach to receptors on other cells and, in the process, transmit the message. Neurotransmitters also trigger, regulate, intensify, or lessen our moods and reactions to situations. In this chapter, I describe the most important neurotransmitters and their nutritional building blocks.

When a few neurotransmitters remain out of balance—their levels are too high or too low—we become susceptible to mood, behavior, or thinking problems. This is because brain cells cannot accurately relay what's going on, leading to responses that are inappropriate to the situation. As a result, depressed people may need to boost their levels of certain stimulating neurotransmitters, whereas hyperactive people might benefit from increasing their calming neurotransmitters. When we don't eat enough of the nutritional building blocks, we reduce our brain's ability to make and properly use neurotransmitters.

Quick Tip

Bad Moods in Perspective
In healthy people, neurotransmitter levels adjust to help us deal with and adapt to changing situations. It's all right to occasionally feel annoyed, angry, or down. These reactions are inappropriate or abnormal only if they occur frequently or are prolonged.

Serotonin is probably the best-known mood-stabilizing neurotransmitter, largely because it is the therapeutic target of several widely advertised antidepressant drugs. Levels of this neurotransmitter are often low in people who exhibit depression, anxiety, and aggressive behavior. Prozac, Zoloft, and several other drugs are frequently prescribed to help the brain maintain higher serotonin levels.

Yet mood disorders do not result from a deficiency of Prozac and Zoloft. Because these drugs are not normal constituents of brain chemistry, they can often strain the biochemical pathways involved in neurotransmitter production. This strain results when certain chemical reactions are artificially sped up, while others remain slow. The situation is somewhat like cooking meat, vegetables, and rice to serve at the same meal. You want all three dishes to be ready at the same time, without one being done earlier or later than the others. Similarly, the timing of a car engine is essential—if the idle is set too high or too low, the engine's performance will suffer.

If drugs were ideal therapeutic solutions, they would rarely produce side effects. Even though Prozac and Zoloft, for example, have helped many people, they often cause low libido in men and women, erectile dysfunction in men, and occasionally suicidal behavior. These drugs modify symptoms of a mood or a behavior problem, but they fail to correct the underlying cause. That cause is usually nutritional and is sometimes due to a combination of nutritional imbalances and genetics.

Neurotransmitters That Calm or Stimulate

Calming Neurotransmitters

These neurotransmitters tend to help you relax and focus, but excessive levels could conceivably leave you feeling oversedated.

- Serotonin
- GABA
- Melatonin
- Nitric oxide

Stimulating Neurotransmitters

These neurotransmitters tend to stimulate your brain, but excessive levels may increase anxiety and wear you down.

- Acetylcholine
- Dopamine
- Norepinephrine
- Epinephrine
- Cortisol
- Phenylethylamine

Neurotransmitters and Neuronutrients

Although a nutritional approach might strike you as being simplistic, it is actually a rational and reasonable way to correct many common mood and behavior problems. For example, nutritionally oriented doctors have used B-complex vitamins for many years to treat a great variety of mood and behavior problems. B vitamins provide some of the building blocks that make neurotransmitters.

Unfortunately, taking vitamins won't fix a bad job or marriage, which might be the psychosocial cause of your moods and behavior. Yet if you support your brain's production of neurotransmitters, they can help you to deal better with difficult situations.

Bill Finds Help for Post-Traumatic Stress Disorder

Bill, who had always been well liked and who had a rewarding job installing air conditioners, returned from a year-long tour of duty in Iraq like a "different person," according to his wife and his employer. His moods seemed to shift from depression to being anxious and jittery. Loud noises made him jumpy, and he frequently had nightmares.

Physicians with the Veterans Administration diagnosed Bill as having post-traumatic stress disorder (PTSD)—he had been in combat, had been shot at, and had seen some of his army buddies wounded or killed. The doctors prescribed drugs, such as Prozac, and recommended psychological counseling. Although Bill's symptoms lessened, they did not go away. His moods and lack of interest in sex were hurting his marriage. At work, customers sensed that something was not right.

A friend suggested that Bill visit a nutritionally oriented naturopathic physician. The doctor recommended a diet emphasizing protein and vegetables, and he asked Bill to avoid soft drinks and fast foods. He recommended that Bill take several natural mood-enhancing supplements, including 5-hydroxytryptophan (5-HTP), gamma aminobutyric acid (GABA), and B vitamins. During this time, the doctor was able to wean Bill from prescription antidepressant and antianxiety drugs.

Bill noticed an improvement within a couple of weeks, and after several months his wife commented that he was more like his old self. The doctor explained that the nutrients helped to restore normal neurotransmitter activity in Bill's brain, leading to more stable moods.

Neurotransmitters That Relax Your Mind

This section covers the most important neurotransmitters, what they do, and the neuronutrients your body needs to make or regulate them. It's important to understand the connection between these neurotransmitters and the neuronutrients in your diet. Your body's production of neurotransmitters depends on what you eat.

Serotonin

What it does. Serotonin is widely considered the principal regulator of good moods, appetite, sleep, and pain. Low levels can result in depression, anxiety, panic disorder, sleeplessness, hunger, insomnia, migraine headaches, obsessive-compulsive behavior, and heightened sensitivity to pain.

Type of neurotransmitter. Calming.

Nutritional building blocks. Serotonin is actually a form of the amino acid L-tryptophan. (Like other amino acids, tryptophan is often written with an "L" prefix.) Amino acids combine to form protein, so you will find L-tryptophan in fish, meats, eggs, and other protein-containing foods. The tryptophan content of protein is one of several reasons why protein-rich foods help to stabilize moods. Vitamin B6 plays a key role in making tryptophan, but vitamins B3 and C are important as well.

The most commonly sold tryptophan supplement is 5-hydroxytryptophan, called 5-HTP. The body quickly converts either 5-HTP or L-tryptophan to serotonin. Inositol, a relative of the B vitamins, can also boost serotonin levels.

Janet Finds Help with Her Alcoholism

Janet began drinking heavily to drown the emotional pain she felt because of her husband's regular affairs. After ten years, she started to attend Alcoholics Anonymous meetings, then filed for divorce. Despite taking concrete steps to deal with her problems, however, she could not always conquer her desire for alcohol, and she had two relapses.

One physician prescribed a drug that was intended to reduce Janet's taste for alcohol, but she stopped taking it because of side effects. She then consulted a nutritionally oriented physician.

This doctor understood that alcoholism was a form of glucose intolerance—that is, a type of prediabetes. He knew that high-sugar diets and cravings for sugary foods often set the stage for alcohol abuse. The doctor recommended a protein-rich diet, containing a lot of chicken and fish, along with high-fiber vegetables to stabilize Janet's blood sugar. He also gave her injections of B vitamins (to speed up their benefits) and vitamin and mineral supplements to be taken with food.

The dietary changes and the extra vitamins and minerals quenched Janet's desire for alcohol; however, she continued to attend Alcoholics Anonymous meetings to reinforce her alcohol-free lifestyle.

GABA

What it does. GABA, short for gamma aminobutyric acid, helps people to maintain mental focus and be relaxed and calm. It promotes good memory, reverses depression, eases anxiety and nervousness, and reduces the sensation of pain. It works by filtering out background noise in the brain. People with anxiety, panic attacks, insomnia, epilepsy, and schizophrenia often have low levels of GABA. Because their minds are not able to filter out extraneous stimulation, they overreact to the excessive sensory input or information, giving other people the impression of being distractible, impulsive, or jumpy.

Type of neurotransmitter. Calming.

Nutritional building blocks. GABA is derived from the amino acid glutamate, with the help of vitamins B3, B6, and B12. (Because glutamate supplements can sometimes stimulate the brain, I don't recommend taking them unless they are prescribed by your physician.) L-theanine, an amino acid found in green tea, boosts GABA levels, and this effect likely explains the calming benefit of green tea. Magnesium stimulates GABA production, and the amino acid L-taurine (another neurotransmitter) also boosts GABA activity.

Quick Tip

If You're Taking Meds for Your Moods, Check with Your Doctor

If you take prescription drugs for depression, anxiety, or another mood issue, work with your doctor before trying natural neuronutrients. Neuronutrients may amplify the drug's effects, and your doctor may need to reduce your medication dosage. Please do not attempt to do this by yourself.

Melatonin

What it does. Melatonin is a hormone and a neurotransmitter secreted by the pineal gland. It regulates our circadian, or daily, body rhythm. Most of us know that we function better and worse at various times of the day, and these differences are related partly to our circadian rhythm. Melatonin levels normally increase toward nightfall, making us sleepy, and decrease toward morning. Taken as a dietary supplement, melatonin can help with sleep disorders and can speed recovery from jet lag, but the timing of supplementation is crucial.

Type of neurotransmitter. Calming.

Nutritional building blocks. Melatonin is made from the amino acid tryptophan and the neurotransmitter serotonin. Its production depends on the same nutrients needed to make serotonin.

How Josh Learned to Chill Out

Josh, whom you met in chapter 1, was totally stressed by work, drove recklessly, and had anger problems. When both his boss and his wife suggested counseling, they were in for a surprise.

Josh's counselor suggested that he adopt several stress-reducing and anger-releasing techniques (which will be described in later chapters). The counselor also recommended that Josh make the time to eat wholesome meals instead of coffee and doughnuts and burgers and fries.

Although Josh was initially perplexed by the dietary advice, he followed through, and his wife began making him high-protein breakfasts before work. Within a couple of days, Josh's mood lightened up considerably. As he practiced the stress- and anger-control techniques, his moods and aggressive behavior continued to improve.

Neurotransmitters That Stimulate Your Mind

Acetylcholine

What it does. Acetylcholine is a key neurotransmitter involved in the thinking processes, memory, motivation, and arousal. Low levels of acetylcholine may interfere with concentration and memory and may lead to emotional instability. Drugs used to treat Alzheimer's disease block the action of an enzyme (cholinesterase) that breaks down acetylcholine in the brain.

Type of neurotransmitter. Mildly stimulating.

Nutritional building blocks. The B vitamin choline lies at the core of this neurotransmitter. Acetylcholine is formed in a chemical reaction with the B vitamin pantothenic acid. Eggs and lecithin are excellent sources of choline.

Dopamine

What it does. Dopamine helps people to focus their attention and enjoy pleasurable physical experiences. It is also involved with physical movement, and people with Parkinson's disease, a neurological disease, have low dopamine levels. In addition, low levels of dopamine are often found in people with sleep disorders, apathy, depression, and increased sensitivity to pain.

Type of neurotransmitter. Usually stimulating, occasionally calming.

Nutritional building blocks. To make L-dopa, the precursor to dopamine, the body uses the amino acid tyrosine, along with folic acid, vitamin B6, magnesium, zinc, and S-adenosyl-L-methionine (a vitaminlike compound also known as SAMe).

Norepinephrine (Noradrenaline)

What it does. Norepinephrine (pronounced nor-ep-uh-neh-frin) plays a key role in fostering upbeat moods, wakefulness, motivation and drive, sexual arousal, learning, and memory. Low norepinephrine levels can be a factor in mood disorders, fatigue, lack of ambition, excessive sleep, depression, and anorexia. High levels can contribute to anxiety, insulin resistance (prediabetes), obesity, feelings of stress, and high blood pressure.

Type of neurotransmitter. Usually stimulating, occasionally calming.

Nutritional building blocks. The basic building block of norepinephrine is the amino acid tyrosine, which is first converted to L-dopa and then to dopamine with the help of folic acid, vitamin B6, magnesium, zinc, and SAMe. Chemical reactions involving vitamins B6 and C and copper convert dopamine to norepinephrine. In addition, the hormone DHEA boosts norepinephrine activity, whereas the stress hormone cortisol inhibits it.

Epinephrine (Adrenaline)

What it does. More commonly known as adrenaline, epinephrine (pronounced ep-uh-neh-frin) is both a stress hormone and a neurotransmitter. When we face danger or stress, epinephrine almost instantly sharpens the mind and prepares the body for a "fight-or-flight" response. Excess adrenaline can be a factor in anxiety, hyperactivity, and feelings of stress. Low levels may result in fatigue, weight gain, poor concentration, and adrenal insufficiency (i.e., weak adrenal glands and a poor response to stress).

Type of neurotransmitter. Stimulating.

Nutritional building blocks. Epinephrine is made from dopamine and norepinephrine, so its production requires the same nutrients as these other neurotransmitters—for example, tyrosine, folic acid, vitamins B6 and C, magnesium, zinc, and copper. The conversion of norepinephrine to epinephrine requires folic acid, vitamin B6, and SAMe.

Cortisol

What it does. Although this hormone is not routinely considered a neurotransmitter, it is so similar to epinephrine that it actually functions as one. Both epinephrine (adrenaline) and cortisol are produced by the adrenal glands in response to stress. Epinephrine is the fast-acting, instant-on stress hormone. When stress is prolonged, such as with daily home and work pressures, adrenaline production decreases and cortisol increases. That's why cortisol is often considered the stress hormone.

Cortisol is highly toxic to brain cells and inhibits the production and growth of new brain cells. Cortisol is often a factor in people who feel anxious without any obvious cause. Some people are particularly prone to extreme stress responses, and they often have short fuses and react with excessive anger to provocations.

Type of neurotransmitter. Stimulating.

Nutritional building blocks. Cortisol has the same nutritional underpinnings as epinephrine. Without extra nutritional support, chronic stress can result in adrenal exhaustion, in which the adrenal glands wear out and can no longer protect against stress. Cortisol also suppresses levels of the hormone DHEA, and low DHEA appears to speed the aging process. In addition, chronically elevated cortisol levels will raise insulin levels, which promote belly fat and abnormal blood sugar fluctuations, as well as increase the risk of diabetes.

How Theresa Quelled Her Anxieties with Equine Therapy

Theresa had been sexually abused as a child and further traumatized in an abusive marriage. Ten years after her divorce, she was still wrestling with severe anxiety, especially in social situations, that medications could not completely resolve.

Theresa entered a clinic that used a mix of counseling, nutritional therapies, and equine therapy—that is, learning to interact with horses. Why horses? Because they seem exceptionally tuned to the moods of people around them and often reflect those moods. For example, a person who is anxious or uncertain will evoke those responses in a horse.

In her first couple of encounters with a horse—petting, walking, brushing, and feeding—Theresa was particularly nervous and worried. After all, a 1,300-pound animal could seriously hurt her, even by accident. Not surprisingly, the horse seemed wary and uncertain. Yet with some tips from the horse trainer, Theresa quickly became comfortable handling the horse, and the horse responded in kind. The experience of interacting with a large animal increased her self-confidence, and her anxieties decreased. Theresa also improved her diet and started taking several supplements, such as 5-HTP and GABA. Together, these methods began to help her overcome the traumas and the anxieties that had shaped her life.

Phenylethylamine

What it does. Phenylethylamine (PEA) is a mood-elevating neurotransmitter that promotes feelings of love and bliss. When relationships end, people often indulge in chocolate, which happens to be high in PEA. Part of the satisfaction of eating chocolate is that it gives the brain feelings similar to those of being in love. If you consume too much PEA, you'll feel anxious and be prone to migraine headaches (a side effect of chocolate for some people). If you have too little PEA, you may feel depressed, tired, and apathetic—often the feelings people have when a romantic relationship ends.

Type of neurotransmitter. Stimulating.

Nutritional building blocks. PEA is built on the amino acid phenylalanine. Chemical reactions involving vitamin B6 convert phenylalanine to PEA. The body can also convert PEA to tyrosine, the building block of dopamine, epinephrine, and norepinephrine. Aspartame, used as a sweetener in soft drinks, is very similar to phenylalanine and may produce edgy feelings.

Other Types of Neurotransmitters and Neurotransmitter-like Substances

Nitric oxide

What it does. Nitric oxide is one of the most versatile neurotransmitters in the brain and in cell-to-cell communication throughout the body. In the brain, it plays a key role in our sense of smell and our ability to form memories. In the rest of the body, nitric acid increases blood-vessel flexibility and regulates blood flow. It dilates (enlarges) blood vessels, lowers blood pressure, and enables men to have erections. Viagra and other drugs that treat erectile dysfunction work by increasing and maintaining nitric oxide levels.

Type of neurotransmitter. Capable of being both calming and stimulating.

Nutritional building blocks. The body makes nitric oxide from the amino acid L-arginine. Supplemental L-arginine increases the body's reservoir of this amino acid, which can then be converted to nitric oxide. L-arginine is the sole precursor to nitric oxide; however, the conversion of L-arginine to nitric oxide requires an enzyme, nitric oxide synthase, that depends on vitamin C.

N-Acetylcysteine

What it does. N-acetylcysteine (NAC) is the standard treatment in hospitals for acetaminophen (Tylenol) overdose and is one of the most effective ways to dissolve mucus in the lungs. It is also a precursor to glutathione, the principal antioxidant made by the body, and helps to protect us from toxic chemicals.

Although NAC is not a true neurotransmitter, it plays a vital role in normal neurotransmitter activity. Cocaine alters the brain activity of glutamate (which is needed for GABA production), and recent studies have found that NAC can restore normal brain levels of glutamate and reduce interest in and desire for cocaine. In a study, cocaine users who took 600 mg of NAC four times daily had a significantly decreased interest in the drug. NAC may also be of benefit in alcoholism and other types of addictions, as well as in obsessive-compulsive and masochistic behavior (e.g., inflicting cuts on oneself).

Type of neurotransmitter. May enhance the activity of a calming neurotransmitter.

Nutritional building blocks. NAC is built around sulfur, and sulfur-rich foods (including garlic, cauliflower, and egg yolk) contain compounds closely related to NAC. Note: Do not take pure L-cysteine unless prescribed by a physician.

How Jessica Learned to Focus

Jessica, whom you met in chapter 1, was addicted to impulsive activities and had difficulty focusing on any single task. Her boss complained about the poor quality of her work, and her distractions led to her being in two fender benders over the previous year.

A friend suggested that she see a nutritionally oriented physician. The doctor diagnosed her with symptoms similar to ADHD (attention-deficit-hyperactivity disorder). After a nutritional workup, he recommended that Jessica take omega-3 fish oils, B-complex vitamins, and an herbal supplement called pycnogenol. Within several weeks, Jessica was better able to focus on single tasks, and her boss noted the improvement in her work quality.

Other Major Influences on Your Moods

Several other key factors influence how you feel. They include glucose, insulin, genetic predispositions, and brain allergies.

Glucose and Insulin: Brain Fuel and Regulator

Although glucose (blood sugar) and insulin are not neurotransmitters, they are essential for normal brain function. Glucose is the principal fuel of brain cells, and insulin regulates glucose levels. The foods you eat influence levels of both glucose and insulin, and their levels affect your moods and your ability to think clearly.

People function at their best when their blood sugar is within a fairly narrow range of glucose levels. The late Emanuel Cheraskin, M.D., D.M.D, noted that people with the "tightest" glucose control (close to 80 mg/dl) were the least likely to suffer from health problems. In general, a healthy range for fasting blood sugar is between 75 and 85 mg/dl, and less than 140 mg/dl after eating.

Doctors have long known that elevated blood sugar levels interfere with concentration, and that poor concentration is often a sign of diabetes. In a recent study, Daniel J. Cox, Ph.D., of the University of Virginia Health System, Charlottesville, confirmed that extremely high glucose levels (270 mg/dl or greater) interfered with normal thinking processes, particularly those related to language and arithmetic. It's likely that more modest elevations can also lead to mental fuzziness and impaired driving ability in some people.

Over the years, many people have attributed their up-and-down moods or postmeal fatigue to hypoglycemia, which literally means "low blood sugar." Conventional physicians have tended to be skeptical of such self-diagnoses of hypoglycemia. The problem, however, is actually not one of low blood sugar so much as it is of either rapid or extreme swings in glucose or insulin levels. Such problems with glucose and insulin are signs of impaired glucose tolerance, prediabetes, or poorly controlled diabetes.

Prediabetes was the focus of my book *Syndrome X: The Complete Nutritional Program to Prevent and Reverse Insulin Resistance.* In the later stages of Syndrome X (a form of prediabetes also known as metabolic syndrome), it's common for people to have both elevated glucose and elevated insulin levels. The body's regulation of glucose goes awry, and it can affect mood, behavior, and thinking processes.

What exactly happens with your glucose and insulin levels?

Eating almost any food leads to a rise in glucose, which in turn prompts the secretion of insulin. Insulin is a hormone that helps move glucose into cells, where it should be burned for energy. Foods rich in protein (e.g., fish, chicken) or fiber (e.g., nonstarchy vegetables, such as broccoli and salad greens) produce only modest increases in glucose and insulin, keeping both within a fairly tight normal range. This is actually why higher-protein, lower-carb diets help people to lose weight—they curb hunger by stabilizing glucose. It's also why they stabilize moods.

Foods that are high in sugars and refined carbohydrates, such as most fast-food meals, convenience foods, and sweets, lead to a rapid and extreme rise in glucose, followed by a surge in insulin levels. During the time that the glucose is elevated (before the insulin has a chance to act), people can lose their ability to concentrate.

Recent research has found that brain chemicals called orexins are responsible for mental alertness. Orexin activity is suppressed by high levels of glucose, leading to poor concentration and sleepiness.

The adage "What goes up must come down" often applies to glucose levels. When glucose levels rise sharply, such as after a high-sugar or high-carb meal, the body's release of insulin can be so strong that it lowers glucose too much, resulting in hypoglycemia—and feelings of hunger, irritability, and physical weakness. People who are sensitive to such changes can experience rapid mood swings, going from calm to angry, upbeat to down. They can also have rapid fluctuations in energy levels, with bursts of energy followed by extreme tiredness. With the preponderance of fast foods and junk foods, more people are eating

How Lynn Found More Energy— and Improved Her Moods

Lynn never seemed to have enough energy. Every day she had to drag herself out of bed and, at night, practically collapsed in bed from fatigue. She snacked on sweets throughout the day, and she swung from being pleasant to irritable. Often her coworkers carefully gauged Lynn's mood before asking her to help out on projects.

Lynn's physician diagnosed her with prediabetes, and he recommended that she follow a high-protein, high-vegetable, low-carb diet. Instead of skipping breakfast, as she usually did, she ate two scrambled or boiled eggs. Within three days of adopting the diet, her energy levels improved—and so did her moods.

foods that are higher in sugars and fats. That's why the incidence of obesity and diabetes has increased rapidly—and part of the reason why I believe mood problems are also on the rise.

Certain Genes Increase the Risk of Depression

Some people inherit genetic and biochemical traits that make them especially susceptible to mood problems. Extreme or chronic stress can aggravate these problems. That's because stress places additional demands on an already weak ability to make or use neurotransmitters.

These genetic traits, which may affect up to half the U.S. population, are known to increase the chances of developing prolonged depression, and similar traits are likely to influence anxiety and other moods. For example, one genetic trait weakens a key enzyme that's involved in making serotonin and other neurotransmitters. Another genetic trait interferes with the transport of serotonin in the brain. Both of these genetic issues increase a person's risk of developing prolonged depression. As I'll explain later, though, supplements of certain neuronutrients can offset these weaknesses.

How Sandy Cured the Blues

In her early fifties, Sandy began to suffer from serious bouts of depression. She lived a high-stress life, running her own business and was always on the go. One doctor prescribed an antidepressant drug, which increased Sandy's weight as a side effect but did not completely resolve her feelings of depression and anxiety. The doctor then prescribed a different antidepressant, but that didn't work well, either.

On the advice of a friend, Sandy visited a nutritionally oriented physician. Blood tests found her low in the B vitamins, so he recommended that she begin taking a high-potency B-complex supplement. Within a week, Sandy's depression and anxiety lifted, and she was able to focus clearly on running her company and enjoying her friends and social activities.

Sandy also reported having a number of side benefits (instead of side effects) from the B vitamins. Her energy levels are higher, and she's sharper mentally. She also lost her sweet tooth, along with twenty pounds in three months.

If you're curious about the effects of genes, nutrition, and psychological stress on physical health, I recommend that you read my book *Feed Your Genes Right* (John Wiley & Sons). Our genes are not our fate—their activity can be modified (positively or negatively) by our eating habits and lifestyles.

Cerebral Allergies Can Affect Your Moods

Physicians who study and treat unusual types of allergies have described what they call "cerebral allergies." It's not clear whether these are true allergies, inasmuch as they don't always provoke the same kind of immune responses that, say, pollen allergies do. Occasionally, however, patients do manifest a reaction to a food or a chemical that is largely limited to mood or behavior.

People with cerebral allergies might be sensitive to any type of food, regardless of whether it's healthful or not, and the allergies may manifest various mental or physical symptoms. In some cases, the symptoms have been described as "brain fog," and at other times, exposure to the problematic food can trigger feelings of sadness and crying.

Because cerebral allergies have not been studied in a scientifically rigorous fashion, it's difficult to say exactly what happens. It is possible, however, that the cerebral allergic reaction causes a leakiness in blood vessel walls, which is common in other types of allergic reactions. In the brain, a slightly leaky blood vessel (far short of what would cause a stroke) could conceivably affect nearby brain tissue.

Often, you can identify food allergies by asking yourself what foods you crave or can't imagine living without. The most likely culprits are foods containing wheat or dairy ingredients.

Basic Neuronutrient Concepts

One basic concept in nutritional therapies and alternative health is that there are many shades of gray—that is, a progression—between health and disease. This is very different from the black-and-white, either/or approach of conventional medicine, in which the absence of any obvious disease is usually considered a state of good health. If you've described your health as "so-so," you know exactly what I mean about being in that vague space between health and disease: you're not sick, but you're not at your best, either.

Recognizing the Spectrum of Moods and Feelings

Most chronic physical diseases develop slowly over many years, following a spectrum of progressively darker shades of gray. For example, heart disease and cancers take years to get to the point of being identified by a physician. It's always easier to prevent a problem or to correct it when it's still in a relatively light (milder) shade of gray rather than a darker (more serious) shade.

The same concept of a spectrum of disease also applies to moods and behavior. The spectrum encompasses a range of behavior, such as irritability to anger to out-of-control rage. Another range of moods would go from your having a sluggish, down day to experiencing normal grief for a few months, to suffering severe and debilitating depression for years.

The Rationale behind Scaling Dosages Up and Down

Another basic concept is that variations in the same nutritional regimen can benefit people who are at any point in the spectrum of moods and feelings. The differences are often in degree—how mild or severe the mood or behavior problems are—and in the dosages of the supplements. For example, what works for irritability will also be effective with more serious forms of anger, except that higher dosages may be needed for the latter.

Conversely, what works for people with serious mood or behavioral problems, such as violent criminal behavior, will often improve less destructive mood problems. Again, the issue is one of dosage. A general rule of thumb is that milder mood and behavior problems usually respond to smaller amounts of supplements. Although vitamins and related supplements are extraordinarily safe, it makes little sense to take higher doses and to spend more money than you need to. Of course, the ideal situation would be to have your levels of vitamins and amino acids measured by a physician, because this approach allows for greater individualization.

None of this obviates the need for psychological counseling. Talk therapies can help people to recognize and change dysfunctional behavior patterns that hurt their relationships at work and at home. Psychological therapies can also reduce feelings of stress, which burn up our calming neurotransmitters. You probably know how good it feels to share (or unload) your personal problems with a trusted friend. Psychological therapy can have similar and greater benefits.

Violence and Nutritional Problems

Studies of criminals, juvenile delinquents, and schoolchildren illustrate certain basic concepts about nutrition, mood, and behavior.

Most of us are concerned by the increase in violence in the world. Violence in prisons, however, is an especially serious problem. After all, people who were violent as free citizens are likely to be violent when they're incarcerated. Yet nutritional supplements and dietary improvements have been found to reduce in-prison violence and rule breaking.

In a study of California inmates, researchers found that prisoners with up to four nutritional deficiencies were 50 percent more likely to be involved in serious violent incidents, and those with five to nine nutrient deficiencies were 90 percent more likely to be involved in violent acts.

Nearly everyone can benefit from either a simple multivitamin or an improvement in eating habits. In a study of eight thousand teenagers at nine juvenile-correction facilities, sociologists arranged to have snack foods that were high in sugar and refined carbohydrates replaced with fruits, vegetables, and whole grains. The change was attributed to budget cuts, so the juveniles didn't realize they were part of an experiment. During the year in which the juveniles' diets were improved, violent and antisocial incidents decreased by almost half. Imagine the benefit to society if at-risk juveniles had enjoyed a nutritious diet all of their lives. Perhaps then they would have had the inner resources to cope with family and environmental stresses instead of acting out in criminal ways.

Until now, I've written mostly about the nutritional and social factors that negatively affect moods. In the next section of *The Food-Mood Solution*, I'm going to describe my four steps to improving your mood.

PART II

How to Improve Your Moods

4

The First Step:
Take Your Supplements

Up to this point, I have focused on how the stresses of contemporary life can negatively affect your nutrition, neurotransmitters, moods, and behavior. In this section of the book, I'll describe four steps you can take to improve your moods and become more stress resistant.

The first step focuses on specific neuronutrients that are essential for improving and stabilizing your moods and behavior. I encourage you to start taking a high-potency multivitamin or B-complex supplement as a general form of mood insurance. Such a supplement will help to jump-start the mood-enhancing, life-balancing benefits of the full program, and you will likely experience positive results within a few days. I'll discuss these nutrients again in part III of the book, in the context of dealing with specific mood and behavior issues.

To simplify the information, I've created a list of twenty different mood and behavior problems and the supplements that can help. (You'll rarely have to take more than two to four of the supplements.) Following the list are several sections that describe the supplements in more detail.

The first group of supplements consists of vitamins, vitaminlike nutrients, and minerals. These neuronutrients are exceptionally safe, and it is virtually impossible to harm yourself with them. The same is true with the second group of supplements, amino acids. With the herbal supplements and hormones, however, it would be prudent to work with a nutritionally oriented physician who has an M.D., a D.O., a D.C., or an N.D. degree.

Supplements Organized by Mood and Behavior Problem

General usage guidelines: Try the first or first two supplements in the category that is relevant to your needs (such as anxiety). If these supplements fail to help or produce only limited benefits after a couple of weeks, then add a couple of others, one by one. If, let's say, the fourth supplement you take yields benefits that the others did not, reduce or eliminate the previous supplements. Without a physician's help you'll need to use trial and error to figure out what works best for you.

Note: If you are taking any medications (Prozac, Zoloft, or others) for mood, do not stop taking them. Work with your doctor during the transition between drugs and nutritional treatments.

Anxiety, Nervousness, and Tension

High-potency B-complex

Vitamin B3

Vitamin B6

Magnesium

GABA

Theanine

5-HTP or tryptophan

Arginine plus lysine

St. John's wort

Sage

Bipolar Disorder

Omega-3 fish oils

High-potency B-complex

Depression

High-potency multivitamin or high-potency B-complex

Vitamin B6

Folic acid (enhances antidepressant drugs)

Inositol

SAMe

Omega-3 fish oils

5-HTP or tryptophan

Tyrosine

St. John's wort

DHEA

Melatonin (for seasonal depression)

Thyroid (with a doctor's prescription)

Depression Plus Overeating

Chromium picolinate

Distractibility

High-potency B-complex

Omega-3 fish oils

GABA

Down Days

Vitamin B12 plus tyrosine

Fatigue

High-potency B-complex

Extra vitamin B1

Vitamin C

Theanine

Fuzzy Thinking or Spaciness

High-potency B-complex

Vitamin B1

Vitamin B12

Omega-3 fish oils

Ginkgo

Impatience

High-potency B-complex

GABA

Theanine

Omega-3 fish oils

Impulsiveness

Omega-3 fish oils

GABA

High-potency B-complex

Magnesium

Irritability, Anger, Aggressiveness

High-potency B-complex or
  multivitamin

Vitamin C

Omega-3 fish oils

Zinc (see chapter 8)

Low Libido

Increase dietary protein, reduce
  sugars and carbs

Arginine

Tyrosine

DHEA (use under a physician's
  guidance)

Memory (Poor)

Phosphatidylserine

Choline or phosphatidylcholine

Omega-3 fish oils

Ginkgo

Ginseng

Migraine Headaches

Vitamin B2

Moodiness

High-potency multivitamin or
  high-potency B-complex

Increase dietary protein, reduce
  sugars and carbs

Obsessive-Compulsive Behavior

High-potency B-complex

Inositol

Dimethylglycine (DMG)

Panic Attacks

High-potency B-complex

Extra inositol

Magnesium

Premenstrual Moodiness

High-potency multivitamin or
   high-potency B-complex

Extra vitamin B6

St. John's wort

Ginkgo

Sleep Problems

GABA

5-HTP or tryptophan

Ginkgo

Ginseng

Melatonin

Stress

High-potency B-complex

Ginseng

Rhodiola

Essential Neuronutrients for Improving Your Mood and Behavior

Action plan: If you are not currently taking any vitamin supplements or a high-potency multivitamin, I recommend that you begin right away. As an alternative, you can also start with a high-potency B-complex supplement. Either of these supplements makes for an excellent foundation for further mood-enhancing supplements. By "high potency," I mean a supplement that contains at least 50 mg each of vitamins B1, B2, B3, and B6. If you get a supplement with 50 mg of these four nutrients, all of the other vitamin levels will pretty much fall into place in terms of their relative dosages. (These amounts are much higher than the government's recommended amounts, but I believe those official amounts are unreasonably low.)

I recommend buying your supplements at health food or natural food stores because their products usually don't contain any sugars or artificial colors. I also list a number of reputable supplement companies in the appendix near the end of the book. By the way, I'm not involved in selling supplements.

Quick Tip

An Important Consideration
If you are taking any psychiatric medications (Prozac, Zoloft, or others), do not stop without consulting your physician or psychiatrist. Tell your doctor that you would like to try some type of nutritional therapy and ask him or her to monitor you during the transition.

Multivitamins

Principal use: To reverse moodiness, irritability, impatience, anger, and depression. Multivitamins are a good all-round mood and mind enhancer.

What else you should know: A high-potency multivitamin (described in the previous section) can have a powerful and positive effect on mood—even if you think you are already even-tempered and normal. This type of supplement will contain most or all of the B-complex vitamins, as well as vitamins C and E and a few other nutrients. It's an ideal supplement for someone who does not want to, or need to, take a lot of capsules or tablets.

Although multivitamins don't have the sex appeal of more exotic supplements, the evidence supports their use, even among apparently healthy people. In one study, David Benton, Ph.D., of the University of Swansea, Wales, asked 127 students to take daily high-potency multivitamins (with amounts about ten times higher than Centrum or One-A-Day) or placebos for one year. After just three months, women taking the multivitamins reported that their moods had substantially improved. These improvements continued throughout the study, and by its end, women taking vitamins reported that they felt more composed, more "agreeable," and in better mental health. Their thinking processes were sharper as well. Men in the study also reported feeling better and more agreeable.

Equally dramatic improvements have been found in children. Bonnie J. Kaplan, Ph.D., of the University of Calgary, Alberta, Canada, and her colleagues described the treatment of eleven children with behavioral disorders, including mood swings, anxiety, obsessive-compulsive disorder, oppositional disorder, bipolar disorder, and Asperger's syndrome. All of the children received a daily high-potency multivitamin/multimineral supplement. After just eight weeks, the children's behavior had gotten significantly better.

Taking a high-potency vitamin supplement is one of the best things we can do for our health, and it's sad that this simple act is so widely ignored or discouraged.

Dosage: Read the fine print on the label to ensure that you're getting

50 mg each of vitamins B1, B2, B3, and B6. If cost is a concern, try a formula with 25 mg each of these B vitamins.

B-Complex Vitamins

Principal use: To reverse moodiness, irritability, impatience, tension, anger, and depression, as well as to increase energy and promote general well-being. It's the best supplement for most people who want to improve or brighten their moods.

What else you should know: This family of eleven related vitamins plays many different roles in making neurotransmitters, burning food for energy, and creating new DNA and cells. Some people benefit from extra amounts of individual B-complex vitamins (see the following sections), which are needed for good moods, thinking, memory, and other brain activities. High doses of any single B vitamin should always be accompanied by either a B-complex supplement or a multivitamin. That's because all of the B vitamins are interdependent.

Dosage: As with multivitamins, read the fine print on the label to ensure that you're getting 50 mg each of vitamins B1, B2, B3, and B6. The potencies of other B vitamins will vary, but they should be fairly consistent between brands. If you want to take individual B vitamins, always take them in addition to a high-potency B-complex or multivitamin supplement. (You most likely do not have to take both a high-potency B-complex and a high-potency multivitamin.)

Vitamin B1

Principal use: To reverse fuzzy thinking and lack of energy.

What else you should know: The University of Wales's David Benton found that a daily supplement of 50 mg of vitamin B1 (also called thiamine) can quickly improve mood. In a study, he asked 120 female college students to take either vitamin B1 or placebos for two months. The women taking vitamin B1 reported feeling more composed, clearheaded, and energetic, and their reaction times sped up as well. All of these improvements occurred even though the women had "normal" vitamin B1 levels when the study began.

Eating large amounts of carbohydrates depletes vitamin B1 levels.

The reason is that a family of enzymes called dehydrogenases helps to break down and use carbohydrates. The body needs vitamin B1 to make these enzymes. So when carb intake is high, your body has to make more dehydrogenases, which means you need more vitamin B1. A diet high in sugars and carbs, however, does not provide that extra vitamin B1.

Dosage: 50 mg daily. Higher amounts may be recommended by a physician.

Vitamin B2

Principal use: For the prevention and reduction of migraine headaches.

What else you should know: Although vitamin B2 (riboflavin) does not have a consistent link to mood problems, it is essential for normal brain chemistry. Low levels of vitamin B2 increase susceptibility to migraine headaches, and, as you might expect, vitamin B2 has been found helpful in reducing the frequency of migraine headaches.

Dosage: To prevent migraine headaches, take 400 mg daily, along with a B-complex supplement.

How Kimberly Regained Her Focus

Kimberly often felt frazzled by the routine activities and demands of life, such as getting her children off to school, arriving at work on time, setting priorities, preparing dinner for her family, and so on. She had difficulty focusing on one task and was easily distracted by telephone calls and e-mails.

A nutritionist suggested that Kimberly start her day with an egg and some fresh fruit, avoid snacking, and have a little more protein and vegetables for lunch (such as a burger without the bun, plus steamed vegetables). The nutritionist also recommended that Kimberly drink a couple of cups of green tea each day—the tea is rich in L-theanine, a natural substance that improves mental focus.

Within a few days of making these changes, Kimberly became less spacey and more focused. She was not as easily distracted or frazzled by what people were doing around her.

Vitamin B3

Principal use: To relieve anxiety. Very large doses may be beneficial for anxiety and cases of acute (recent onset) schizophrenia.

What else you should know: In the early 1950s, the Canadian psychiatrist Abram Hoffer, M.D., Ph.D., and his colleagues began to treat schizophrenic patients with relatively high doses of vitamin B3 (niacin or niacinamide) and vitamin C. They theorized that schizophrenics were genetically predisposed to making their own hallucinogen, a by-product of adrenaline called adrenochrome. Hoffer and his associates conducted the first double-blind studies in psychiatry and published their results in the prestigious *Bulletin of the Menninger Clinic*. Hoffer's work has never been accepted by mainstream medicine, partly because much of medicine has a bias for pharmaceuticals over inexpensive vitamins.

Vitamin B3 is a powerful mood-enhancing nutrient, and it is involved in the chemical reactions that make the calming neurotransmitter serotonin. There are two common forms of vitamin B3: niacin and niacinamide.

The niacin form, which also lowers cholesterol, causes an intense tingling and a flush that lasts for about one hour. It feels like an allergic reaction, although it seems to bother some people less than others. I mention this reaction because people who take niacin may be frightened by the flush if they don't anticipate it. Some people actually like it because it increases circulation to the hands and the legs, resulting in a warming sensation. The niacinamide form of vitamin B3 does not cause this flush, nor does it lower cholesterol levels.

I recommend against taking time-release niacin supplements. These supplements are more likely than ordinary niacin to raise liver enzyme levels, which may indicate problems with normal liver function.

Dosage: For schizophrenia, take 3,000 mg of vitamin B3 and 3,000 mg of vitamin C daily. You can get the cholesterol-lowering effect of niacin (not niacinamide) by taking 1,000 mg daily.

Vitamin B6

Principal use: To reduce irritability, anxiety, tension, depression, premenstrual mood changes, and a "climbing the walls" feeling.

What else you should know: Vitamin B6 (also called pyridoxine and pyridoxyl-5-phosphate) may be the single most important B vitamin in terms of mood and behavior. B6 works with folate, vitamin B12, and tryptophan to make serotonin. As you read in chapter 3, low serotonin levels can cause a variety of mood problems, including depression, anxiety, panic attacks, and obsessive-compulsive disorders.

One benefit of vitamin B6 is in treating the physical and behavioral symptoms of premenstrual syndrome (PMS). PMS is akin to having a bad mood for several days each month, and, in some women, symptoms may include depression, irritability, anxiety, tension, and aggressiveness. In an analysis of nine studies in which vitamin B6 was used to treat PMS, researchers reported that the vitamin reduced overall symptoms by more than half.

Some people are genetically predisposed to producing large amounts of kryptopyrrole when stressed. Kryptopyrrole increases the excretion of vitamin B6 and zinc, reducing serotonin production and the creation of new brain cells. Not dreaming or not being able to remember your dreams is a sign of vitamin B6 deficiency, and white spots on the fingernails are a sign of zinc deficiency.

Dosage: Take 50 to 250 mg daily, plus a B-complex supplement. If you take more than 100 mg of vitamin B6 daily for longer than six months, ask your physician to measure both your vitamin B6 and your aspartate aminotransferase levels. The latter is an enzyme that depends on vitamin B6, and low levels indicate poor vitamin B6 activity.

Folate (Folic Acid)

Principal use: It's involved in serotonin production and will enhance the activity of antidepressant medications.

What else you should know: This B vitamin is crucial in the production of neurotransmitters and brain cells. Folic acid supplements can enhance the benefits of antidepressant medications. This shouldn't be surprising because folate contributes to the body's production of serotonin. Inadequate intake of folic acid has been found to boost the risk of Alzheimer's disease.

Dosage: Take 400 mcg to 5 grams daily. Always take it with vitamin

B12, with the B12 dose being half that of the folic acid. Because folate enhances the effects of antidepressant medications, you will likely need a lower dose of those drugs, which is good.

Randy Finds a Solution for Violent Behavior

Randy had been a problem child. When he was three years old, he was stepping on insects and at age four killed the family's pet cat. He expressed absolutely no remorse to his parents (whom he threatened to kill), and psychological therapy failed to improve his behavior. By age fourteen, after being arrested for fighting, he was incarcerated in a residential facility for violent juveniles.

Although officials were skeptical, they allowed Randy's parents to have him evaluated at a nutritional medicine center. Doctors found high levels of lead and copper, along with low zinc levels, in his blood—a combination that could affect his behavior. The center customized a nutritional supplement regimen for Randy's particular needs, and he was permitted to take the supplements during his incarceration.

Over the next two months, Randy's behavior improved significantly. He became more athletic, had fewer violent thoughts, and had no scuffles with other people. At the end of the third month, Randy was symptom free and was allowed to return home and to school, where his grades became better than average. His behavior at home and school substantially improved, and he showed no signs of violence or sadism.

Vitamin B12

Principal use: To promote mental sharpness and clarity.

What else you should know: Low intake of vitamin B12 is strongly associated with severe depression. In addition, deficiencies of vitamin B12 can sometimes mimic symptoms of severe brain fog and Alzheimer's disease. Because vitamin B12 is relatively inexpensive, everyone who is suspected of having Alzheimer's or another type of dementia should be tested for his or her levels of vitamin B12 and methylmalonic acid, which reflect vitamin B12 activity. Some people may have normal vitamin B12 levels but abnormal methylmalonic acid levels.

Approximately one-third of senior citizens suffer from atrophic gastritis, a condition in which they don't produce enough stomach acid. A lack of stomach acid interferes with the absorption of vitamin B12. Like folic acid, vitamin B12 is involved in the production of DNA, which is needed to make new brain cells.

Drugs such as omeprazole (Prilosec), which reduce gastric acid secretion, also lower B12 absorption. In addition, antacids, antibiotics, oral contraceptives, and the use of nitrous oxide anesthesia during surgery can reduce B12 levels.

Recent studies have found that sublingual (under the tongue) vitamin B12 tablets increase blood levels just as well as injections do. As the sublingual vitamin B12 dissolves, it enters a network of blood vessels located under the tongue. If you are deficient in vitamin B12, however, you may need several hundred times the recommended daily amount to restore normal blood levels of the vitamin. That amount translates to 600 to 1,000 mcg of vitamin B12 daily.

Dosage: Take 500 to 1,000 mcg daily.

Choline and Phosphatidylcholine

Principal use: To improve memory.

What else you should know: Choline is a B vitamin that plays a major and usually underrecognized role in mood and brain function. It is a component of acetylcholine, a neurotransmitter that is necessary to thinking and memory. Animal experiments have shown that prenatal choline supplements improve the brain function of offspring.

Choline is also part of phosphatidylcholine, a type of fat needed by brain cells. Lecithin, a supplement derived from soybeans, is about one-fourth phosphatidylcholine. The best form of lecithin is in granules, which have a slight nutty flavor and can be sprinkled on cereal or simply chewed by the tablespoonful. Lecithin capsules contain much smaller amounts of phosphatidylcholine.

Dosage: Take 250 to 1,000 mg of choline or one heaping tablespoon of lecithin.

Inositol

Principal use: For depression, anxiety, panic attacks, and obsessive-compulsive disorder.

What else you should know: Chemically speaking, inositol is related to glucose, but it's not a sugar. Functionally, it's a distant relative of the B-complex family that is involved in maintaining normal neurotransmitter levels and DNA production.

Several clinical studies have found large amounts of inositol to be highly effective in reducing symptoms of depression, panic attacks, and obsessive-compulsive disorder. In these studies, the dosages ranged from 12 to 18 grams a day, which, unfortunately, amounts to a lot of tablets or capsules. Despite all of the inositol pills that had to be taken in these studies, the supplement is far safer than drugs given for the same disorders.

Dosage: Twelve to 18 grams of inositol can add up to a lot of capsules or tablets, and I empathize with people who prefer to take as few pills as possible. I believe that many people can achieve the same benefits by

Quick Tip

Mellow Out with Mood-Boosting Aromas

The basic ideas behind aromatherapy have been part of religion, traditional medicine, and cosmetics for hundreds of years. Does what we smell actually affect our moods? Of course! After all, we generally find that perfumes and colognes make a person more sensual and sexually attractive.

There is a difference, however, between aromatherapy and perfumes. Aromatherapy is based on natural essential oils extracted from plants, whereas perfumes and fragrances are usually made from synthetic molecules created in a laboratory. As potent as natural essential oils are, their effect can be greatly enhanced by using them to lubricate the skin during a therapeutic massage.

Researchers have determined that the scent of lavender increases alpha waves in the brain, which is the type of brain activity associated with relaxation, and jasmine increases stimulating beta waves. So if you want to calm down, expose yourself to lavender, and if you want to sharpen your mind and senses, opt for jasmine.

Mindy Green, an aromatherapist and educator in Minneapolis, Minnesota, recommends a blend of several essential oils for reducing stress. This blend, which you can buy at most natural foods stores, includes 5 drops of lavender, 3 drops of chamomile, 2 drops of bergamot, and 2 drops of clary sage, combined together in 1 ounce of a carrier oil or lotion. You can use this blend in a bath, as a body lotion, or to keep in a small vial to sniff when you find yourself in a stressful situation.

combining 3 to 4 grams of inositol with a high-potency B-complex supplement.

SAMe

Principal use: To reduce depression and pain (especially osteoarthritis).

What else you should know: SAMe, technically known as S-adenosyl-methionine, is the key product of what biochemists call the SAM cycle. SAMe is formed by chemical reactions involving folic acid, vitamins B6 and B12, and choline, and it feeds into one of the most remarkable and diverse molecule-building processes in the body. The end products include DNA, neurotransmitters, and phospholipids—the latter being specialized fats needed for normal brain function.

SAMe is an excellent treatment for depression and osteoarthritis. Although these two conditions seem totally unrelated to each other, they both depend on SAMe's molecule-building activities. SAMe supplements can help to regenerate joint cartilage and relieve joint pain. They are also highly effective in reducing depression. Both the pain-relieving and the antidepressant effects are related to increases in serotonin.

The major drawback to SAMe is its cost. It's very expensive, as over-the-counter supplements go, and for this reason I usually recommend first trying a high-potency B-complex supplement and perhaps extra vitamin B6. If this approach fails, then try SAMe for one month to see if it might help.

Dosage: Take 400 to 800 mg twice daily.

Vitamin C

Principal use: To ease irritability and fatigue. It may enhance the activity of antipsychotic drugs.

What else you should know: Many physicians assume that patients have an adequate intake of vitamin C unless they have symptoms of scurvy, the classic deficiency disease in which blood oozes from old wounds as the body literally disintegrates. Negligible amounts of vitamin C will prevent scurvy, which actually describes the final stage of deficiency before death. Mark Levine, M.D., Ph.D., a researcher at the U.S. National Institutes of Health, has found that the first symptoms of vitamin C deprivation are actually irritability and fatigue, two very common conditions.

Vitamin C has numerous roles in brain chemistry. The brain contains the highest concentration of vitamin C of any organ in the body, with levels up to 25 times higher than those in the blood. It is essential for the conversion of dopamine to norepinephrine, and it protects against toxicity from high levels of some neurotransmitters. Vitamin C also enhances the activity of certain antipsychotic drugs, while protecting the brain against amphetamines.

Dosage: Take 1,000 to 10,000 mg daily. Divide the dosage, so that you take it two or three times daily. If you develop diarrhea, you're taking too much. Ignore statements warning that the body cannot use more than 200 mg of vitamin C daily. That paltry recommendation was based on a study of healthy college-age young men, and the researchers acknowledged that it did not apply to women, middle-aged or older people, or those suffering from health problems.

Chromium

Principal use: To reverse depression, particularly when it involves overeating. It can lower and stabilize insulin and blood sugar levels, which may lessen mood swings.

What else you should know: Chromium has long been recognized for its essential role in regulating insulin and glucose in the body. Until just a few years ago, no one could have imagined that it could reverse feelings of depression, reduce appetite, and help in some eating disorders.

Malcolm McLeod, M.D., a psychiatrist at the University of North Carolina School of Medicine, Chapel Hill, became curious when patients taking medications for depression and overeating suddenly felt better, ate less, and lost weight after they started taking supplements of chromium picolinate. Rather than dismiss his patients' testimonials, McLeod tested chromium picolinate supplements on other patients. Many were able to reduce or eliminate their prescription antidepression medications. Chromium may increase brain levels of tryptophan and serotonin.

Dosage: Take 400 to 1,000 mcg daily. Divide the dosage, so that you take half the amount twice a day.

Magnesium

Principal use: To reduce nervousness, anxiety, jittery feelings, agitation, twitchiness, and muscle spasms. It may have some benefits in post-traumatic depression and anxiety.

What else you should know: Magnesium plays a role in more than three hundred enzymatic reactions in the body, influencing heart rate, muscle tone, bone density, labor, and the risk of headaches. Muscle spasms, charley horses, and restless legs syndrome are often signs of magnesium deficiency.

The mineral is essential for relaxing muscles. Your heart is a muscle, and it pumps blood by repeatedly contracting and relaxing. Its contraction depends in part on calcium, whereas relaxation requires magnesium. The same principle applies to other muscles in the body.

French researchers found that a combination of magnesium and vitamin B6 supplements reduced hyperactive symptoms in children. Those symptoms included poor attention, physical aggressiveness, twitchiness, and spasms. Adults with similar problems will also benefit from magnesium along with B-complex vitamins.

Dosage: Take 400 mg of magnesium citrate daily. Higher doses may loosen bowels or cause diarrhea, although the risk can be reduced by splitting the dosage so that you take 400 mg in the morning and 200 to 400 mg later in the day.

Omega-3 Fish Oils

Principal use: To relieve depression, bipolar disorder, poor memory, impulsiveness, hostility, and physical aggressiveness, and improve thinking processes.

What else you should know: The omega-3s are among the most healthful of all dietary fats. They are needed for normal brain development in infants and children and for normal brain function in adults. Omega-3s are found in salad greens, flaxseed, grass-fed meats, and coldwater fish, such as salmon. Fish are the preferred source because the omega-3s exist in more biologically active forms, specifically eicosapentaenoic acid (EPA) and docosahexaenoic acid (DHA).

EPA and DHA are incorporated into the fatty membranes (walls) of cells, where they influence how cells communicate with each other. When other fats are incorporated in their place, communication between brain cells is disrupted.

In ancient times, people consumed roughly equal amounts of the omega-3s and the omega-6s and no trans fats. Today, the average American eats twenty to thirty times more omega-6s than omega-3s, as well as substantial amounts of trans fats. As a result, the omega-3s are virtually nonexistent in many people's diets, contributing to depression and other mood disorders. High intake of the omega-6s increases the risk of depression, whereas many studies have found that omega-3 fish oil supplements are helpful in treating depression. They also function as a mild blood thinner and a regulator of heart rhythm.

Other studies have found that the omega-3s can help to reduce impulsive behavior, hostility, and physical aggressiveness. In a double-blind study of forty middle-aged men and women, taking 1.5 grams of DHA daily led to significant reductions in aggressive behavior toward other people in just two months. It's noteworthy that hostility and physical aggressiveness are strongly associated with an increased risk of heart disease, and the omega-3s are also well documented for reducing this risk.

Dosage: Take 3 to 10 grams daily, either in capsule form (3 to 10 capsules) or by the tablespoon. Some brands of liquid fish oils, such as those from Carlson Laboratories (800-323-4141), have a lemon taste that makes them more palatable than other brands.

Phosphatidylserine

Principal use: For memory, especially age-related memory decline.

What else you should know: Serine is an amino acid, and phosphatidylserine is a fatty substance found in the brain that incorporates serine into its structure. Phosphatidylserine is incorporated into the fatty membranes (walls) of brain cells, where they maintain a youthful flexibility and enable communication between brain cells. Supplements have been found to blunt the release of cortisol, a stress hormone. In a study of young adults, taking 300 mg of phosphatidylserine daily for one month led to fewer feelings of stress, better moods, and less neurotic behavior.

Phosphatidylserine has also been shown to improve memory and to reverse age-related memory loss. In one of several studies, Thomas H. Crook, Ph.D., a clinical psychologist in Scottsdale, Arizona, gave 300 mg of phosphatidylserine daily to 149 patients with age-related memory impairment. After twelve weeks, patients taking phosphatidylserine scored about 30 percent better in terms of learning and recalling names, faces, and numbers, compared with people taking placebos.

Dosage: To optimize cognitive function, take 100 mg of phosphatidylserine one to three times daily.

Protein and Individual Amino Acids That Improve Mood and Behavior

Action plan: Protein consists of amino acids, which are the building blocks of neurotransmitters, so it's important to eat high-quality protein, such as fish, chicken, and turkey. In general, individual amino acid supplements are best taken on an empty stomach, ten to twenty minutes before breakfast and one hour away from eating food at any other time of day.

Protein

Principal use: To stabilize mood swings.

What else you should know: Protein has gotten a bad rap because of widespread misunderstandings about high-protein, low-carbohydrate diets. It is an essential nutrient, and there are many low-fat sources of animal protein, including chicken, turkey, and fish. (Vegetarians can focus on legumes, eggs, and dairy products for protein.) Extreme high-protein, zero-carb diets were recommended by the late Robert Atkins, M.D., but for only a short period of time, after which carbohydrate intake could be increased. My dietary recommendations (in chapter 5) can best be described as protein rich, relatively low in fat, with substantial amounts of vegetables and small amounts of carbohydrate.

High-quality protein stabilizes blood sugar levels. In people with elevated blood sugar, protein generally lowers and steadies their blood sugar levels. This dampens hunger, which in turn reduces appetite and often leads to weight loss. The effect of protein on blood sugar is rapid.

Eating a high-protein breakfast, such as eggs, results in improved blood sugar levels and fewer feelings of hunger by lunchtime.

Dosage: It is a good practice to eat a little high-quality protein with every meal, when you feel that your mood is deteriorating, or when you need a mental energy boost. One of the fastest ways to improve your mood is to eat some protein, such as a couple of slices of deli turkey and cheese.

Arginine

Principal use: To treat anxiety and erectile dysfunction.

What else you should know: Arginine (also known as L-arginine) is the immediate precursor to nitric acid, a neurotransmitter that can lessen anxiety, restore blood vessel tone, and improve erectile function. A recent study found that a combination of 3 grams of arginine and 3 grams of lysine (another amino acid) daily reduced anxiety in high-strung people.

Dosage: For anxiety, try 1 gram of arginine three times daily. If this doesn't help, add 1 gram of lysine three times daily. Follow the same dosage for erectile dysfunction, but consider taking one dose about thirty to sixty minutes before intercourse. Always take arginine at least one hour before or after eating any food.

GABA

Principal use: For anxiety, distractibility, and difficulty sleeping.

What else you should know: GABA, or gamma aminobutyric acid, is an amino acid that also functions as a neurotransmitter. It's one of the best brain-calming supplements. Conventional psychiatrists sometimes use a related compound to treat anxiety, but it's far more straightforward and less expensive to use GABA.

Researchers only recently discovered one of the key ways in which GABA relaxes the mind. GABA helps to filter out background noise in the brain. By allowing the brain to process only the most important and relevant information, GABA actually improved how elderly monkeys responded to visual images. In fact, their improvement was so great that their brains registered visual images just as well as those of young monkeys did. This may account for why GABA can sharpen the mind at the same time that it relaxes it.

Dosage: Like other amino acids, GABA works best when taken on an empty stomach, such as about twenty minutes before eating or drinking anything (except water) for breakfast, before bedtime, or at least two hours apart from eating any food. The reason is that other amino acids in food can interfere with the absorption of GABA. Take 500 to 600 mg one to three times daily, and consider combining it with 200 mg of theanine.

Glycine and Dimethylglycine

Principal use: For obsessive-compulsive behavior and blood sugar regulation.

What else you should know: Dimethylglycine (DMG) is used in the SAM cycle (see SAMe, earlier) and is the precursor to glycine. Glycine is the simplest amino acid in chemical structure and functions as an inhibitory, or calming, neurotransmitter. It has many other roles in the body, such as protecting cells from toxins and reducing inflammation.

Research conducted at the University of Minnesota, Minneapolis, found that glycine supplements could significantly lessen the postmeal rise in blood sugar levels, which would help to prevent diabetes and mood swings.

DMG specifically has been used with vitamin B6 and magnesium to alleviate symptoms of autism. In two case reports, DMG decreased obsessive-compulsive behavior in autistic men.

Dosage: To control blood sugar levels, take 3 to 5 grams of glycine daily with meals. For obsessive-compulsive behavior, try 300 to 400 mg of DMG daily, but cut the amount if hyperactive behavior increases.

Theanine

Principal use: For difficulty relaxing, anxiety, tension, and poor mental focus.

What else you should know: Theanine (known as L-theanine) is an amino acid found in green and black teas. It accounts for the taste of tea, and higher-quality (and generally more expensive) teas have higher concentrations of theanine. Theanine improves mood by increasing levels of serotonin, dopamine, and GABA. The result is a sharpening of mental activities, along with a mild tranquilizing, anxiety-reducing effect. Some reports describe the effect as being similar to meditation.

Theanine increases the activity of alpha waves in the brain, which researchers have long known to be associated with feeling relaxed and alert—in effect, mellow and perceptive. According to an article by Raymond Cooper, Ph.D., in the *Journal of Alternative and Complementary Medicine*, people with high alpha-wave brain activity are less anxious, and creative people produce more alpha waves when trying to solve a problem.

The theanine concentration in tea may explain the beverage's soothing effects. In fact, some research suggests that theanine counteracts the edginess of caffeine, which is also found in tea. However, this caffeine-moderating effect does not seem to work consistently with everyone.

Dosage: Theanine supplements are sold in health food stores. Dosages range from 50 to 200 mg, taken one to three times daily. When you shop, look for the "SunTheanine" logo on the bottle, which indicates a high-quality source. You can safely combine it with GABA, and some formulations do combine them. Based on research, GABA starts relaxing the mind thirty to forty minutes after ingestion. Another option is to drink one or two cups of green tea daily.

Tryptophan and 5-hydroxy-tryptophan (5-HTP)

Principal use: For depression, anxiety, and insomnia.

What else you should know: The amino acid tryptophan (also known as L-tryptophan) is the precursor to serotonin, and serotonin is really just a more biologically active form of tryptophan. It has a powerful calming, antianxiety, and antidepressant effect. Low intake of tryptophan reduces serotonin production and activity in the brain.

Tryptophan is available by prescription, although a few companies do sell it over the counter. More readily available over the counter is 5-hydroxytryptophan, also known as 5-HTP, which is the immediate precursor to serotonin.

Dosage: For anxiety, depression, or restless sleep, take 50 to 200 mg of 5-HTP daily, with the last dosage about thirty to sixty minutes before bedtime. For tryptophan, take 500 to 3,000 mg before bed. With either form of the supplement, start with the lower end of the dosage range.

Tyrosine

Principal use: To treat depression or occasional down feelings.

What else you should know: Tyrosine (also known as L-tyrosine) is an amino acid and a precursor for the neurotransmitters norepinephrine and dopamine. In high doses, it can help to treat some cases of depression. It may be particularly beneficial for people who lack motivation and drive, have poor sexual arousal, and sleep excessively.

Nearly everyone has occasional down days, in which they temporarily feel—often for inexplicable reasons—a little depressed. A low dose of tyrosine, along with vitamin B12, can often lift this mood within an hour or two.

Dosage: For the occasional down day, take 500 mg of tyrosine and 500 mcg of sublingual vitamin B12 with water and at least twenty minutes before consuming any other beverage or food in the morning. For more serious and prolonged depression, try 500 to 3,500 mg in the morning, at least twenty minutes before eating. It's all right to take a second dose midafternoon without food.

Herbs That Improve Mood and Behavior

Action plan: Herbs contain hundreds of natural ingredients, some of which have nutritional activity and others that are similar to certain prescription medications. Although herbal remedies are generally safe, they may increase or decrease the activity of prescription drugs you might also be taking. If you find yourself taking more than four to six supplements without experiencing clear benefits, it's time to start working with a nutritionally oriented physician. You'll find ways to locate a nutritional physician in the appendix. Don't be reluctant to spend the money—your improved well-being will be worth every penny.

St. John's Wort

Principal use: To relieve mild to moderate depression, although it may be of some help with severe depression and anxiety and premenstrual syndrome.

What else you should know: Although occasional news reports and medical journal articles try to dismiss the benefits of St. John's wort (*Hypericum perforatum*), the herb is one of the most effective treatments for mild to moderate depression. In high dosages, it might also help in severe depression.

The scientific evidence supporting the use of St. John's wort for depression is extensive and persuasive. In direct comparisons, researchers have consistently found that it works just as well as, if not better than, conventional prescription treatments for depression. For example, studies have found that St. John's wort has better results than Prozac (fluoxetine) and Zoloft (sertraline) and is equal to Tofranil (imipramine) in treating mild to moderate depression. The herb was also more effective than Paxil (paraxetine) in treating severe depression and better than Tofranil in reducing anxiety. Furthermore, St. John's wort causes few side effects compared with drugs. Drug side effects include reduced interest in sex and erectile dysfunction in men—which, ironically, are reasons to feel depressed! Occasionally, taking these drugs will lead to an increase in suicidal thoughts and behavior.

St. John's wort is widely used to treat depression in Europe, where herbs have been used medicinally for at least two thousand years, but the U.S. pharmaceutical industry has convinced most American physicians that its higher-priced drugs are superior. The herb can also help to alleviate symptoms of premenstrual syndrome, including anxiety, depression, nervous tension, confusion, and crying.

Dosage: The chemical constituents of St. John's wort will vary between batches, so shop for a standardized product. (This will be identified and explained on the label.) For depression, take 300 mg three times daily. If this dosage fails to help after one month, try doubling it for several weeks. On rare occasions, St. John's wort may increase eye and skin sensitivity to sunlight. It will also improve liver function so that medications (including oral contraceptives and chemotherapeutic agents) break down faster and may be less effective.

Note: Work with your physician if you want to transition from an antidepressant drug to St. John's wort. Do not combine St. John's wort with any antidepressant drugs except under the guidance of your doctor.

Ginkgo

Principal use: For memory, mental function, and premenstrual symptoms.

What else you should know: Ginkgo (*Ginkgo biloba*) is a venerable Chinese herb whose benefits in mental function are now being confirmed by scientific studies. Fuzzy thinking can impair judgment, and poor memory can contribute to feelings of frustration and anxiety.

Studies have shown that ginkgo supplements increase blood circulation in the brain and activate brain activity. In an animal study, researchers found that ginkgo extracts boosted the activity of ten essential genes in brain cells by up to sixteen times. One of the genes influenced the hippocampus, the brain's center of learning and memory. The other nine genes affected the cerebral cortex, which controls memory, speech, logical and emotional responses, and voluntary physical movements. Another gene influenced the activity of tyrosine, the amino acid precursor to norepinephrine and dopamine. In a British study, researchers gave college students either 240 or 360 mg of ginkgo extracts or placebos. The students' memories and the speed of their thinking processes improved after taking ginkgo.

Researchers at Oregon Health Sciences University, Portland, found that ginkgo extracts improved various thinking processes in patients with multiple sclerosis. The subjects experienced an improvement in attention, planning, and decision making. All of the patients had previously sustained cognitive impairments as part of their multiple sclerosis.

Dosage: Take 240 to 360 mg of standardized ginkgo extract daily. Divide the amounts, and take them two or three times daily.

Ginseng

Principal use: For memory and adapting to stress.

What else you should know: Several different species of herbs are called ginseng, and all of them function as "adaptogens," or substances that help people adapt to stressful situations. Adaptogens are useful, but it's important to find other long-term ways of reducing stress in your life.

When we're chronically stressed, our memory often becomes worse. High levels of the stress hormone cortisol interfere with memory and the production of new brain cells. Ginseng supplements can buffer some of that stress, at least temporarily.

British researchers tested whether combined extracts of ginkgo and ginseng (*Panax ginseng*) would improve memory in healthy middle-aged men and women. The dosages were either 60 mg of ginkgo extract and 100 mg of a standardized ginseng extract twice daily, 120 mg of ginkgo and 200 mg of ginseng in one daily dose, or placebos. The researchers reported in the journal *Psychopharmacology* that the people taking the herbs "were remembering more information than those taking placebo."

Dosage: Take 100 to 200 mg of a standardized ginseng extract daily.

Rhodiola

Principal use: For chronic stress.

What else you should know: Rhodiola (*Rhodiola rosea*) is considered an adaptogen and has been reported to be helpful in preparing for and weathering physical, mental, and emotional stresses. It appears to work by reducing the breakdown of serotonin, dopamine, and norepinephrine.

Like the adaptogenic herb ginseng, rhodiola is probably best used for relatively short periods, such as weeks or months rather than years, as an interim means of bolstering resistance to stress. It makes far more sense to avoid long-term stresses.

Dosage: Use a rhodiola product that has been standardized to a consistent level of rosavin, a key compound found in the herb. Rosavin concentrations generally are 1, 2, or 3.6 percent. For 1 percent standardized rosavin, take 360 to 600 mg of rhodiola daily. For 2 percent standardized rosavin, take 180 to 300 mg of rhodiola daily. For 3.6 percent standardized rosavin, take 100 to 170 mg daily.

Sage

Principal use: To treat anxiety and restlessness.

What else you should know: Common sage (*Salvia officinalis*) is a culinary herb and is often used as a rub on chicken and turkey. A close botanical relative known as Spanish sage (*S. lavandulaefolia*) has smaller leaves but a stronger flavor and aroma. Spanish sage can also improve mood and memory.

In a study conducted in England, Andrew B. Scholey, Ph.D., and his colleagues asked twenty-four healthy male and female students to take capsules containing a small amount of oils extracted from Spanish sage. The herbal extract improved memory, but the most significant response was in mood. After taking the sage extract, the subjects felt more alert, calm, and contented, and the benefits lasted for several hours afterward.

Dosage: For supplements, follow the label directions regarding dosage. For cooking, mince sage or use whole leaves to season chicken or turkey.

Hormones That Improve Mood and Behavior

Action plan: Hormones have a powerful effect on neurotransmitters, and they should be used only with the guidance of a physician. Your physician can test your blood levels of DHEA and thyroid hormone to determine whether they are normal or low. You will need a prescription for thyroid hormone; DHEA and melatonin can be purchased without a prescription.

DHEA

Principal use: For moderately severe depression, lack of sexual desire, and erectile dysfunction.

What else you should know: DHEA (dehydroepiandrosterone) is a steroid hormone and a precursor to estrogen and testosterone. In the mid-1990s, it became a popular over-the-counter supplement because it could improve muscle tone, enhance sexual desire and performance, and increase general feelings of well-being. The drawback is that it can be abused by people who have normal hormone levels, and it could conceivably increase the risk of estrogen-dependent and testosterone-dependent cancers.

That said, DHEA may help moderately severe depression. If you want to try DHEA, have your DHEA-S levels measured by your doctor and follow his or her guidelines for use. In a recent study, researchers found that high doses of DHEA relieved depression in elderly men and women and led to improvements in arousal, orgasm, and other aspects of sexual activity.

Dosage: When it comes to DHEA, follow your doctor's advice. If your DHEA levels are low, you may need only 25 to 50 mg daily when combined with B-complex vitamins. Your doctor might also recommend a high dose for several weeks to rapidly boost your hormone levels, followed by a much lower maintenance dose.

Melatonin

Principal use: For difficulty sleeping, restless sleep, insomnia, jet lag, and seasonal depression.

What else you should know: Melatonin, when used correctly, is one of nature's best sleep aids. It is a hormone and a neurotransmitter that regulates our circadian, or daily, body rhythm. Normally, melatonin levels increase toward evening and make us drowsy, then decrease toward morning. Too much time indoors and under artificial light, however, seems to throw off normal melatonin production. People who suffer from seasonal depression, usually during the winter, often benefit from melatonin supplements.

Dosage: Melatonin supplements are sold without a prescription, but the effective dosage varies greatly among people. For example, one-quarter milligram (0.25 mg) works for me (when I've needed to take it), while some friends need a whopping 9 mg. Taking too little will be ineffective, whereas too much will probably leave you feeling sluggish the next day.

The timing of its use is critical. For sleep problems or seasonal depression, take melatonin one to two hours before bedtime. Do not drive after taking melatonin. To reduce jet lag, start taking melatonin a day or two before you travel, about one to two hours before you would go to sleep in the new time zone.

Thyroid Drugs

Principal use: To treat depression, lack of energy, or weight gain, particularly among women between the ages of forty-five and sixty.

What else you should know: Thyroid hormone typically refers to two hormones: T3 and T4. During perimenopause, thyroid hormone levels may decrease along with estrogen levels. It's often difficult to accurately measure T3 and T4 levels because of natural shifts in hormone levels. Sometimes a physician will base a diagnosis on clinical symptoms, such as those described in the previous paragraph.

Although low thyroid activity (hypothyroid) is not a common cause of depression, it could be a factor, particularly in middle-aged women. It's important, however, to consider whether lifestyle issues, such as self-esteem and changing physical appearance, might be causing depression.

As medications go, thyroid drugs are relatively inexpensive, about $12 per month. You may discover that your biggest argument with a doctor will be about the type of thyroid medication you take. He or she may want to prescribe Levoxyl, Synthroid, Levothyroid, Euthyrox, or a generic levothyroxine. Insist that your doctor at least initially prescribe Armour thyroid (produced from the thyroid glands of pigs). It's the most natural of thyroid drugs and provides both T3 and T4. (The others provide only synthetic T4.)

Dosage: Follow the dosage advice of your physician or pharmacist.

How Liz Dealt with Depression

Liz, a successful artist and writer, was in her midthirties when feelings of severe depression turned her life upside-down. Antidepressant medications didn't help, and she came close to committing suicide.

She kept thinking that low thyroid might have something to do with her symptoms. She lived in the Southwest, but she never sweated. Thyroid tests showed her levels of thyroid hormones to be in the normal range. Meanwhile, Liz said that her energy level was low and she felt as weak as an old woman.

Liz finally found a doctor who was willing to give her a trial prescription of a moderate dose of thyroid hormone. Twenty minutes after taking the first pill, she said, she began to sweat. She considered that a validation of her gut feeling about having low thyroid activity.

In less than a month, she had regained her energy levels and enthusiasm for life. Liz's depression had vanished. Twenty years later, in her midfifties, Liz maintains a work schedule and a vibrancy that her younger colleagues have trouble matching. She's also still taking thyroid hormone.

5

The Second Step:
Eat Mood-Enhancing Foods

Nutritional supplements and lifestyle improvements go a long way toward providing and preserving the neuronutrients you need to promote healthy moods and behavior. Eating healthy foods, however, will complete the nutritional circle of my four-step program.

As impressive as the benefits of supplements are, their full results are realized only when combined with dietary changes. Sound eating habits provide a strong foundation for optimal brain chemistry, whereas supplements strengthen specific biochemical processes that affect mood and behavior.

In this chapter, I describe my dietary guidelines, offer sample recipes, and outline a two-week menu plan. I recommend that you eat mostly nutrient-dense foods—by doing so, you will consume the highest concentration of good nutrition per bite or calorie. The alternative, which is not desirable, is eating calorie-dense foods that are high in sugar or simple carbohydrate starches, without any redeeming nutritional value.

My dietary guidelines refine and simplify those in my previous books, including *Feed Your Genes Right*, *The Inflammation Syndrome*, and *Syndrome X*. Here, I describe my guidelines in practical terms and with only a brief explanation of the rationale behind them. If you would like a more in-depth discussion, please refer to my previous books.

The recipes illustrate healthy cooking and eating. You may not have time to make complicated meals, so many of the recipes are simple and quick to prepare. Others are more complicated and can be made on weekends when you have time to experiment and be creative in the kitchen. Feel free to adjust ingredients, such as spices, to suit your personal taste.

The two-week menu plan consists of meals that you can cook at home or eat in restaurants. You don't have to follow a rigid plan. Instead, treat the menu as a list of options from which you can choose healthy meals to suit your tastes and schedule.

Discover the Joy of Cooking

Cooking is more than preparing a meal. It can be one of the most creative, fun, and satisfying experiences in life. The meal, if you prepare it with fresh and wholesome ingredients, benefits your overall physical health, replenishes your neuronutrients, and feeds your neurotransmitters. Both the process of cooking and the end product (which you get to eat!) are good for your mood.

I now enjoy cooking, but I didn't always relish being in the kitchen. Until 1999, I rarely cooked for myself, and my forays into the kitchen were usually to be served or to heat a packaged meal in the microwave oven. When I found myself living alone (after my divorce), I learned how to cook in a series of baby steps, sometimes by observing or assisting friends in the kitchen and other times by watching chefs on the Food Network.

Despite the popularity of cookbooks and celebrity chefs, cooking often seems to be a dying art. Many people, especially women, feel that cooking is drudgery. Such feelings typically result from having to cook for other people, making uninspired meals, or simply being too rushed or tired to enjoy the experience of preparing fresh foods.

I believe the situation has been made worse by overprocessed convenience and fast foods, which have dulled our palates to what good food really tastes like. As a result, eating becomes an exercise in quickly satisfying our hunger instead of turning on our senses of sight, smell, and taste.

There is (at least to me) a boring sameness when it comes to the greasy smell and taste of fast foods. Overprocessing has ruined many traditional tasty foods. Consider the modern tomato, which is picked green (so it can be shipped without bruising) and sprayed with ethylene gas to turn it red. The tomato never really ripens, and it tastes like pulp. Or, consider the most widely marketed Thanksgiving turkey, which is so heavily treated that it has an artificial, chemical-like taste. It's enough to kill a hearty appetite, along with the desire to cook.

Cooking can be a meditative experience in which you quietly appreciate cutting up and preparing food. Working in the kitchen can be like a group of musicians jamming together, starting with a recipe and then spontaneously improvising. It can be playful and even sensual. If food often equates with love, then making food can be a prelude to making love. On that note, you can treat meal preparation as a form of culinary foreplay, or you can make it a fast-food quickie.

Once you begin to make the lifestyle changes I recommend in chapter 7, you will have time to cook. Consider cooking at home an investment in your neuronutrients and neurotransmitters. Nutritious foods lay a foundation for long-term health, whereas supplements jump-start and fine-tune your brain chemistry.

My Ten Guidelines for Mood-Enhancing Eating Habits

Guideline 1. Eat a Little Protein at Each Meal

Here's why: Protein stabilizes blood sugar, lessens appetite, and reduces the amount of food you subsequently consume. More stable blood sugar levels protect you from mood swings and fatigue. By helping to control appetite, protein will promote weight loss and reduce your risk of developing diabetes. Just as important, protein provides many of the molecules, such as L-tryptophan, GABA, and L-tyrosine, that your body needs to make neurotransmitters. You don't have to go on a so-called high-protein diet. Rather, think of your eating habits being protein rich. If you are taking antidepressant medications, such as Prozac or Zoloft, they will work better if you eat a little more protein.

Examples: Fish, chicken, turkey, and eggs are excellent sources of protein; however, don't have deep-fried protein, such as deep-fried fish or chicken. You can also eat certain deli meats, such as turkey and chicken; fresh-cut deli meats (Applegate Farms, Boar's Head, and Diestel are good brands) are usually healthier than prepackaged brands.

If you are a vegetarian, opt for eggs, cheese, sugar-free yogurt, hard European cheeses (from animals not given growth hormones), and legumes. Be aware, however, that allergies to dairy and soy are common, and legumes have relatively large amounts of carbohydrates. If you are a vegetarian and are overweight, or you suffer from mood problems, your current diet may not be ideal for you.

> **Quick Tip**
>
> **Always Eat Breakfast**
> Several studies have found that eating a low-glycemic breakfast—that is, high in protein or high-fiber foods—improves a person's overall blood sugar level by lunchtime. It can also reduce your appetite and the amount of food you eat throughout the day.

Guideline 2. Eat a Variety of High-Fiber Nonstarchy Vegetables

Here's why: Fiber helps to stabilize blood sugar, again protecting you from mood swings. Fiber also helps to move food through your digestive tract, so you're less likely to be constipated—that's important because being regular also helps your moods! The foods highest in fiber are usually those that have little starch and sugar, so there's a double benefit from eating them.

Examples: High-fiber nonstarchy vegetables include most fresh salad ingredients, such as dark lettuces (Romaine, bibb), spinach, arugula, tomatoes, cucumbers, mushrooms, red bell peppers, and onions. Other high-fiber nonstarchy vegetables include asparagus, broccoli, carrots, cauliflower, green beans, kale, leeks, and shallots, all of which can be prepared in a variety of ways. Fresh is better than frozen, and both fresh and frozen vegetables are far superior to canned.

Guideline 3. Eat a Variety of High-Fiber Nonstarchy Fruits

Here's why: Some research has shown that diets high in vegetables are healthier than those high in fruit. My hunch is that the nutritional value of highly cultivated fruits is often diminished by their sugar content. Still, many fruits are relatively low in sugars and very healthful.

Examples: Fresh raspberries and blueberries are at the top of my list of healthy fruits. You can use frozen but unsweetened berries if they are out of season or if cost is a limitation. Don't buy canned fruits because they almost always have added sugars. I also like fresh apples, kiwifruit, cantaloupe, honeydew, watermelon, and the occasional banana or pear. (Bananas and pears have been cultivated for high sugar content.) The same is true of citrus. Occasional citrus fruit is fine, but avoid drinking orange juice, which provides a lot of sugars without any fiber.

Guideline 4. Cook with Olive Oil or Macadamia Nut Oil

Here's why: Both olive oil and macadamia nut oil are rich in oleic acid, which is anti-inflammatory. Stress triggers a low-grade inflammatory response, which these oils can help to protect against. They might also ease some of your aches and pains.

Examples: Extra-virgin olive oil has the greatest nutritional value, but other types of olive oil are better for cooking at high temperatures. Macadamia nut oil has a more neutral flavor, despite a subtle nutty aroma. It also has a very high smoke point (the temperature at which oil smokes or burns), making it better to use when sautéing or stir-frying at high temperatures. You can occasionally use canola oil, which is sometimes substituted for olive oil in processed foods.

Guideline 5. Drink Water and Teas

Here's why: When we're thirsty, our bodies are signaling that they want water. Yet many people quench their thirst with coffee, juices, or soft drinks that contain large amounts of sugar, caffeine, or both. Diet soft drinks also have their downsides: the artificial sweetener aspartame is closely related to a stimulating neurotransmitter, which may contribute to impulsive or hyper behavior, and phosphoric acid reduces bone density. The caffeine in coffee (and in many soft drinks, such as Coke, Pepsi, Red Bull, SoBe No Fear, Full Throttle, Monster, and Mountain Dew) can contribute to impatience and irritability.

Examples: Water might seem a bit boring, but a wedge of lemon, lime, or orange can make it more interesting to your palate. Mineral waters, especially European brands, have appreciable amounts of calcium and magnesium, which are good for the body and mind. Green, black, and white teas contain caffeine (less than coffee, though), but the effect of the caffeine is often neutralized by their L-theanine content.

A variety of health food brand herbal teas, such as those made by Celestial Seasonings and Stash, make tasty hot and iced caffeine-free teas. You can make sun tea by allowing two to three teabags to brew for several hours in a quart pitcher of water in the sun—or on your kitchen counter. One or two cups of weak home-brewed (or watered-down) coffee daily are probably all right for many people.

Yet another beverage option is a veggie drink, such as Greens8000, which contains very few calories. (It's sweetened with the herb stevia, which has no calories.) All you have to do is mix a little into a glass of cold water. (See ordering information in the appendix.)

Guideline 6.   Avoid Fast-Food and Chain Restaurants

Here's why: With few exceptions, these restaurants serve up everything that's bad for you: foods rich in refined carbohydrates, sugars, and the unhealthiest fats. These foods could be labeled "obesity in a bag" or "diabetes in a bag" because they contribute so much to the risk of obesity and diabetes. As an example, numerous studies have found that McDonald's meals negatively alter blood vessel function and blood flow. That's bad for your heart and your head—after all, your brain depends on a steady supply of blood. If you're not seduced by the smell of burgers, fries, and other cooked foods, you might choose something from the salad bar, only to end up using a salad dressing loaded with unhealthy fats and sugars.

Examples: McDonald's, Burger King, Wendy's, KFC, Taco Bell, Carl's Jr., and Denny's, are among the many fast-food and chain restaurants to avoid.

Guideline 7.   In All Restaurants, Practice Defensive Eating

Here's why: It is possible to navigate menus in most restaurants, but the guiding rule is this: don't assume anything about what will be served on your plate. A meal such as a chicken Caesar salad that is usually similar from one restaurant to another may be very different in the restaurant you've chosen. Not making assumptions means that you will ask a lot of questions, so don't be shy about it. For example, you'll want to ask whether the restaurant adds croutons, a refined carbohydrate, to its salads. If it does, ask the waiter to leave them off.

Examples: You'll generally have better luck at many ethnic restaurants, particularly Greek, Middle Eastern, Japanese, and some Italian restaurants. Seafood and upscale new American cuisine restaurants usually offer healthy meals, but you must be a responsible consumer and ask questions before ordering. Follow guidelines 1, 2, and 5 when ordering.

The key is to avoid starchy foods (such as pasta, white rice, or potatoes), deep-fried foods (such as fries or falafel), and the breadbasket. (Ask the waiter to take it back the moment he or she brings it.) Greek, Middle Eastern, and Italian restaurants typically use olive oil to cook with, and you will do best ordering chicken, fish, meats, and vegetables. The new American cuisine tends to be very inventive and typically uses high-quality ingredients in preparing fish, chicken, and other dishes, although it can sometimes be pricey. A baked or rotisserie half-chicken is usually a tasty and moderately priced meal.

Guideline 8. At Home or the Office, Avoid Prepackaged Microwave Meals

Here's why: It's certainly fine for you to reheat home-cooked meals in a microwave oven, but nearly all of the microwavable meals sold in

Quick Tip

Read the Fine Print

There ought to be a sign warning "Let the Buyer Beware" when you walk into supermarkets. Most foods sold in a jar, bottle, box, or plastic bag contain less-than-healthy ingredients. And those unhealthy ingredients add up. A few grams of sugar here and a few grams there turn into 150 pounds of sugar each year for the average American.

The key to being a defensive supermarket shopper is to read the fine print on the back of the package, particularly the nutrition information box and the list of ingredients. Here's where you'll discover trans fats, partially hydrogenated vegetable oils, high-fructose corn syrup, and other ingredients you want to avoid.

At first, you'll find it difficult (though not impossible) to avoid unhealthy ingredients. You'll have better luck at natural foods markets and specialty grocers, but even here you should never assume that a packaged food contains only healthy ingredients. For example, dried cranberries are usually sweetened, and some brands of "natural" yogurt contain trans fats.

packages contain far too much in the way of sugars, refined carbohydrates, unhealthy fats, or chemicals that enhance their appearance or taste.

Examples: Microwave meals are designed by food technologists to survive cooking, freezing, and microwaving. They're more of a testament to technology than to good nutrition. Nearly all brands leave a lot to be desired, but you may be a little better off with Indian- or Thai-style meals, if you like those cuisines. Be just as circumspect when looking at the fine print of health food brands.

Guideline 9. Avoid Most Refined Oils

Here's why: Olive oil, macadamia nut oil, and avocado oil are healthy, but most other oils are not. The worst offender is trans fat, found in shortening and often disguised under the term *partially hydrogenated vegetable oils*. It's equally important to avoid corn, soybean, and peanut oils, which are all high in inflammation-promoting compounds that promote damaging stress responses.

Examples: Nearly all fried foods are cooked in a blend of unhealthy oils, including trans fats. Heating increases the amount of trans fat, sometimes up to 40 percent of the oil. French fries and chicken nuggets are saturated with these awful fats. So are almost all of the bakery products made in supermarkets, nondairy creamers, nondairy whipped creams, and many other products.

Assume that all cooked foods in fast-food and other chain restaurants use large amounts of these unhealthy oils. Any packaged food that lists "partially hydrogenated" vegetable oils also contains trans fats. Furthermore, be aware that trans fats don't have to be listed on a label if there is less than one-half gram per serving—a "gotcha" because people commonly eat more than one serving at a meal. Incredible as it might sound, trans fats are far more hazardous than saturated fats.

Guideline 10. Avoid or Strictly Limit Your Intake of Sugars and Grain-Based Carbohydrates

Here's why: Eating foods that contain sugars (such as sucrose and high-fructose corn syrup) destabilizes blood sugar levels, increases the risk of diabetes, and contributes to mood and behavior problems. There's some evidence that large amounts of fructose—what you get in processed foods but not in fruit—actually alters the brain centers involved in regulating appetite.

When grains, such as wheat and corn, are refined, food particle size is reduced through grinding, and fiber is either similarly reduced in size or removed altogether. The result is a wheat- or corn-containing food that is absorbed almost as quickly as pure sugar.

Examples: Sugars, such as sucrose and high-fructose corn syrup, are found in nearly all nonfruit sweets, including desserts, doughnuts, pastries, and muffins, as well as soft drinks. Refined grains are used to make bagels, breads, pastas, and pizzas—and most whole-grain breads and pastas are also problematic. They are still highly refined, though not quite as bad as white breads or pseudo whole wheat breads (that is, white breads with molasses added to darken their color).

Main Courses for Dinner

Sautéed Chicken Breast   (Serves 2)

2 half chicken breasts, boneless and skinless
1 teaspoon extra-virgin olive oil
1 pat butter
sea salt
fresh ground black pepper
sauce (optional, to add at last minute)

Prepare the chicken breasts either by cutting them laterally so they are only about half as thick or by flattening them with a food mallet. To flatten the breasts, place them in a large sealed plastic bag or wrap them in wax paper with the edges securely folded over. Then pound them until they are flat and thin.

Heat a 10- or 12-inch nonstick skillet over medium-high heat. When the pan is hot, add the olive oil and melt the butter, swirling it around the pan. When the butter bubbles and sizzles, add the chicken breasts and cook them for about 2 or 3 minutes. Sprinkle them with salt and pepper, then turn them over and cook them for another 2 or 3 minutes. If the breasts are thick, they will take longer to cook. If you want the chicken to cook a little faster, cover the pan to retain moisture and heat. (Aluminum foil will work if you don't have an actual cover.)

Sautéed Chicken Breast *(continued)*

As the chicken cooks, it should turn white. If you are unsure about whether it is cooked through, cut it through the middle; it should be white and juicy, not yellow or pink. When the chicken has about a minute left to cook, add the sauce, if desired (see my sauce recipes). Serve the chicken breast as is, or reserve it for another meal, such as my Quick-and-Easy Caesar Salad (see page 121).

Coated and Sautéed Chicken Breast   (Serves 2)

1–2 eggs
1–2 chicken breasts, boneless and skinless
1 cup Lotus Foods' Bhutanese Red Rice Flour*

In a medium-size bowl, whisk the eggs. After cutting or pounding the breasts, dip them in the egg and dredge them in the red rice flour. The egg and flour coating helps to seal in moisture while the chicken cooks; it browns nicely and adds a wonderful flavor. Follow the cooking instructions for Sautéed Chicken Breast on page 95.

Chicken Piccata   (Serves 4)

This meal takes a little longer to prepare, but the result is incredibly flavorful. Try it on a weekend when you have time to spare.

1 to 1½ pounds chicken breasts or chicken tenders, boneless, skinless
¼ cup Lotus Foods' Bhutanese Red Rice Flour* or brown rice flour
¼ teaspoon paprika
extra-virgin olive oil
butter
2 garlic cloves, minced
1 medium-size shallot, diced
4 fresh sage leaves, minced; or 1 teaspoon dried sage
½ cup extra-dry vermouth or very dry white wine
1 cup high-quality chicken broth (such as Pacific brand)
2–3 tablespoons small capers, drained
juice from 1 lemon
lemon slices and parsley (optional)

*This can be ordered at www.lotusfoods.com.

Slice the chicken breasts horizontally, then wrap them in plastic and pound them with a food mallet to flatten and tenderize them. If you're using chicken tenders, slice them to remove the silvery membrane and discard it.

On a shallow plate, spread about ¼ cup of red rice flour or brown rice flour. Add ¼ teaspoon of paprika and mix it into the flour with your finger. Roll the chicken pieces in the flour to coat them.

Heat a deep covered nonstick frying pan over medium-high heat. When it's hot, add 1 tablespoon of olive oil and 1 tablespoon of butter. Swirl the butter around the pan until it melts and sizzles, then add the chicken. Cook the chicken for 1 to 2 minutes, then flip over the chicken pieces and cook them for another minute.

With tongs or a slotted spoon, remove the chicken. Add a pat of butter and a small amount of olive oil to the pan. When the butter melts, add the garlic, shallot, and sage, allowing them to sauté for about a minute or so.

Add the vermouth, letting it boil off for about 30 seconds; then add the chicken broth and capers. Add about half of the lemon juice. Allow the sauce to reduce by one-third to one-half. (The alcohol in the vermouth will evaporate during the cooking.) Put the chicken into the pan, add the rest of the lemon juice, and let it simmer with the cover on for another 1 or 2 minutes. Garnish with lemon slices and parsley.

Sautéed Shrimp   (Serves 3)

2 tablespoons extra-virgin olive oil
1 pat butter
4 garlic cloves, minced
1 large shallot, diced
1 pound large shrimp, tail on or off, uncooked, deveined
1 teaspoon or so dried basil
1 teaspoon or so dried oregano
juice from 1 lemon

Heat a large nonstick frying pan or a wok over medium-high heat. When it's hot, add the olive oil and butter. When the butter melts, swirl the oil and butter around to cover the bottom of the pan. Sauté the garlic and shallots until they're soft, 1 to 2 minutes. Next, add the shrimp, then the

Sautéed Shrimp *(continued)*

basil and oregano. After about a minute, turn the shrimp over or move them around with a heat-resistant spatula. When the shrimp turn pink, they are ready to eat. Squeeze the lemon juice over the shrimp and serve.

Alternative: Try the dish with my Mustard-Garlic Sauce (see page 108), in which case you will still use the garlic, but not the shallot, basil, or oregano. Add the mustard sauce at the time when you would have added the spices.

Shrimp and Scallop Pesto with Jasmine Rice   (Serves 2–4)

1 cup jasmine brown or white rice
2 scallions
1 small carrot
1 tablespoon extra-virgin olive oil
1 pat butter
2 tablespoons pine nuts
6–10 medium to large shrimp, cut in 1-inch-long pieces
12–20 small bay scallops
2 pesto cubes, defrosted (see Traditional Pesto Sauce recipe, page 107)

Cook the jasmine rice, timing it to be ready a few minutes before the shrimp and scallops. While the rice is cooking, dice the scallions and finely slice the carrot with a vegetable peeler.

Heat a frying pan over medium-high heat, then add the olive oil and butter. When the butter sizzles, add the scallions and carrot and sauté for about 1 minute. Add the pine nuts and continue sautéing for another minute. Add the shrimp and scallops and sauté for 3 to 4 minutes, until the shrimp turn slightly pink and the scallops white.

Add the jasmine rice and pesto to the wok and mix everything with a spatula until the seafood is dispersed and the rice absorbs some of the pesto. Serve the dish immediately or reheat it in the microwave for a later meal.

Pan-Fried Salmon   (Serves 1)

1 salmon fillet, about the size of your hand and ½- to ¾-inch thick
dried basil, to taste
dried oregano, to taste
1 teaspoon extra-virgin olive oil

Rinse the fillet under cold water and pat it dry with a paper towel. Sprinkle a little basil and oregano on the fleshy (nonskin) side of the fillet. Heat a nonstick frying pan over medium-high heat. When the pan is hot, add the olive oil. (Salmon is oily, so you won't need as much olive oil as you might with other types of fish.) When the oil is hot, after about a minute, place the salmon fillet in the pan, skin-side up. Cook it for about 3 minutes. Turn the fillet over and cook it for another 3 minutes.

Roast Chicken   (Serves 3–4)

For this recipe, you will need a roasting pan with a removable wire rack. The chicken will rest on the rack while the pan catches the drippings that you will use for the gravy.

1 4-pound whole chicken
4–5 garlic cloves, minced or sliced
leaves from several sprigs fresh rosemary, chopped
1 cup high-quality chicken broth (such as Pacific brand)
½ cup filtered water

Preheat the oven to 425 degrees F. Remove the chicken from its plastic or paper wrapping. Remove and discard the giblets, which will have been inserted into the cavity and wrapped in waxed paper. Rinse the chicken inside and out under cold running water. Pat it dry with paper towels and place the chicken, breast-side up, on the wire rack in a roasting pan. With your fingers, loosen the skin located above the breast to create a pocket. With a small knife, cut through the skin over the thighs to make two more small pockets. Insert the garlic and rosemary into the pockets. Put any extra rosemary and garlic inside the stomach cavity.

Roast the chicken for about 1 hour. Use an instant-read thermometer to determine that the meat in the thickest part of the breast is 160 to 165 degrees F. If it isn't that hot yet, continue cooking the chicken for a few

Roast Chicken (continued)

more minutes. A larger chicken will need about 10 minutes of additional cooking time per pound of weight. When it's done, transfer the chicken to a serving plate and allow it to rest for 10 minutes to redistribute its juices.

Meanwhile, place the roasting pan (without the rack) over medium heat. Add the chicken broth and water. Bring it to a boil. With a wooden spatula, scrape the bottom of the pan to loosen the brown bits. Allow the gravy to reduce by about half, stirring occasionally. Taste and season it with a little salt, if desired. Pour the gravy over slices of the chicken.

Alternative: Instead of rosemary and garlic, use a combination of garlic and sage or a combination of tarragon, coarse Dijon mustard, and lemon juice.

Note: After serving the chicken, you will probably have leftovers. Remove most of the chicken from the bone and use the remaining carcass to make Chicken Rice Soup (see below).

Chicken Rice Soup   (Serves 4)

For this recipe, you'll need a stockpot at least 7 or 8 inches high and roomy enough for the leftover chicken bones and carcass. You'll also want several plastic containers to freeze the soup for later use.

leftover chicken and bones from previous recipe
1 medium-size red or sweet onion, diced
3 stalks celery, diced
2–3 large carrots, cleaned and sliced
1 teaspoon dried thyme
1 teaspoon fresh ground black pepper
2 bay leaves
filtered water
1 cup cooked brown rice

Remove and discard all of the visible skin from the chicken and place the bones in the stock pot. Add the onion, celery, carrots, thyme, ground pepper, and bay leaves. Fill the pot with just enough water to cover the chicken. Bring the water to a boil, place the cover a little ajar so that some of the water can evaporate, then reduce the heat to a simmer for 2½ to 3 hours. Turn off the heat, cover the pot tightly, and allow it to cool. When it's cool, place the covered pot in the refrigerator overnight.

The next day, use a large spoon to skim the fat off the top of the liquid. Remove the breast bone and leg bones, pull off any edible meat from the bones, putting the meat back into the soup, and then discard the bones. Sift through the soup looking for small bones and joints that might have fallen off and discard them.

Place a small amount of cooked brown rice in 3 or 4 plastic containers. With a ladle, transfer some soup to each container, but don't fill them all the way to the top. (The volume will expand a little when you freeze the soup.) Seal the containers and freeze them for future use.

At least partially defrost the chicken soup before heating it in a pot. Salt it to taste.

Seared Ahi Tuna   (Serves 2)

Wasabi horseradish paste or Terrapin Ridge Wasabi Squeeze*
3 tablespoons tamari or light soy sauce
1 teaspoon macadamia nut oil
2 slices sushi-grade ahi tuna, ½- to ¾-inch thick
shredded cabbage or store-bought cole slaw mix

Prepare the wasabi sauce a few minutes before searing the tuna. Do this by mixing a small amount of wasabi horseradish paste with 3 tablespoons of tamari or light soy sauce. Alternatively, you can mix about 1 teaspoon of Terrapin Ridge Wasabi Squeeze with 3 tablespoons of tamari or light soy sauce. Be careful with the concentration of wasabi because it can be very hot!

Rinse the tuna under cold water and pat it dry. Heat a large nonstick frying pan over high heat and add the nut oil. When the oil is hot, place the tuna in the pan. Allow it to sear for no more than 30 seconds. While it is searing on the first side, spread a little wasabi sauce on the tuna, then sear the other side. Serve it on a bed of shredded cabbage. Use the rest of the wasabi sauce for dipping.

*This can be ordered at www.terrapinridge.com.

Braised Beef Brisket (Serves 4)

Braising is a method of slow cooking in a small amount of liquid that's well suited to tough but ultimately tasty cuts of meat. The prep for this meal takes about 15 minutes; then it cooks in the oven for about 3 hours. You'll need a Dutch oven—a deep oval-shaped glass or metal cooking pot with a tight-fitting cover.

2–4 tablespoons extra-virgin olive oil
1 beef brisket, 3–5 pounds
1 large red or other type of sweet onion, sliced
10 garlic cloves, minced
¼ cup red wine or balsamic vinegar
2 cups high-quality beef or chicken broth (such as Pacific brand)
1 teaspoon dried basil
2 teaspoons dried oregano

Heat the Dutch oven over medium-high heat on the stove top and add 2 tablespoons of olive oil. When the oil is hot, place the brisket in the Dutch oven, fatty-side down, and sear it for 3 minutes. Keep the Dutch oven covered as much as you can while searing the brisket. Turn the brisket over and sear the other side, then remove it and set it on a plate for a few minutes.

Sauté the onions and garlic in a little olive oil until they're fairly soft. Add the vinegar, followed by the broth. Stir in the basil and oregano and mix together any bits of beef or fat that were left on the bottom of the Dutch oven. With a large spoon, move the onion and garlic to the side and place the brisket back in the Dutch oven; spoon the onions and garlic over the brisket.

Cover the Dutch oven and place it in the oven, which should be preheated to 325 degrees F, for 1 hour. Reduce the heat to 300 degrees F and continue baking for another 2 hours. After about 2½ hours of baking, use an instant-read food thermometer to check the interior temperature of the thickest part of the brisket. It's safe to eat if it's at least 145 degrees F (rare). Cook it until it's 160 degrees F if you would like it more well done.

When the brisket is cooked to your personal taste, transfer it to a serving plate, cover it with aluminum foil, and allow it to rest for 10 minutes. It will continue to cook from its own heat. Cut *against* the grain of the meat. (The direction of the grain will be obvious.) Spread some of the onion-garlic mix with the gravy over the meat.

You can also refrigerate the brisket overnight, which will firm up the meat and make it easier to cut. Slice it thinly and store it in a sealed container.

Tip: If you store the gravy, separate the onions and garlic and store them in a another container. When the gravy is refrigerated, the fat will rise to the top. You can discard this. To reheat the brisket, lay several slices on a plate, spread some of the onion-garlic mix and gravy on top, then cover it loosely with wax paper and place it in a microwave oven.

Pan Fried and Steamed Dumplings   (Serves 1–4)

You can buy frozen Asian-style dumplings at Trader Joe's and many other specialty food stores. They are similar to the gyoza or dim-sum you'll find at restaurants. The ingredients aren't perfect—there is, after all, the refined carbohydrate shell that wraps around the chicken, pork, or shrimp. Still, unless you're sensitive to wheat or must strictly limit your carbohydrates, you can have these dumplings occasionally. They cook fairly quickly in a pan, steamer, or microwave oven.

I prefer to cook them in a large nonstick frying pan. The key is to pre-pare the dipping sauce (see the following recipe) a day earlier. Although the dipping sauce is tasty when fresh, the flavors integrate and strengthen when the sauce has been refrigerated for a day or two.

1 tablespoon macadamia nut oil
10 dumplings per person, frozen
$\frac{1}{8}$ cup water
shredded cabbage or store-bought bag cole slaw mix
Chinese Dipping Sauce (see the next recipe)

Heat 1 tablespoon of macadamia nut oil in a large nonstick frying pan over medium-high heat. Add the dumplings, crinkle-side up. Cook them

Pan Fried and Steamed Dumplings *(continued)*

for about 2 minutes or until they brown slightly. Add the water and cover the pan. (Aluminum foil is fine if you don't have a cover, but always use the shiny side against the food. The dull side has a plastic coating.) Reduce the heat to medium and continue cooking the dumplings for about 8 more minutes. Meanwhile, spread some of the cabbage on a dinner plate. When the dumplings are cooked, place them on top of the cabbage. Spoon some sauce on top of the dumplings and pour the rest into a small dish to use for dipping.

Chinese Dipping Sauce   (for previous recipe)

Use this sauce cold or at room temperature for dipping Pan Fried and Steamed Dumplings (see previous recipe), Seared Ahi Tuna (see page 101), or other firm fish.

¼ cup tamari or low-sodium soy sauce
¼ cup oyster sauce (available at Asian markets)
⅜ cup rice cooking wine (mirin, available at Asian markets)
1 tablespoon sesame oil
1 heaping tablespoon fresh ginger root, peeled and finely minced
2–4 cloves fresh garlic, finely minced
1 teaspoon honey
¼ teaspoon red chile powder

Combine the tamari or low-sodium soy sauce, oyster sauce, rice wine, and sesame oil in a 2-cup measuring glass or bowl. Add the ginger, garlic, honey, and red chile powder. Stir to mix all the ingredients together. You can use the dipping sauce immediately, but the flavors develop more if the sauce is refrigerated overnight.

Exotic Red Rice Dinner Crepes and Pancakes   (Serves 4)

Working with rice flour can be a little less predictable than with wheat flour, but even if these crepes happen to fall apart, the pieces have an amazing taste.

1 cup Lotus Foods' Bhutanese Red Rice Flour*
2 tablespoons cornstarch, mixed with 3 tablespoons water
½ teaspoon honey
½ teaspoon sea salt
½ cup light coconut milk
¾ cup filtered or distilled water
2 whole eggs

Mix all of the ingredients together in a large bowl and whisk them by hand to blend. Heat an 8- or 10-inch nonstick frying pan over medium-high heat. When it's hot, pour some of the crepe batter into the center of the pan. You'll have to eyeball the right amount—the batter will start to solidify within seconds, so work quickly to spread the batter by tipping the pan. Cook the first side for 2 to 3 minutes, then carefully flip the crepe over, and cook the other side for another 2 minutes.

For a filling, use a sauce-rich leftover, such as brisket or sautéed shrimp. Cut the filling into small pieces and heat it in a microwave oven while the crepe is cooking. When the crepe is done, transfer it to a dinner plate. Spoon the filling in a line across the center of the crepe. Fold over one third of the crepe, put a small amount of the filling on top of the first fold, then fold over the other side. Serve it immediately.

Alternative: You can also use Forbidden Rice Flour, distributed by Lotus Foods.

*This can be ordered at www.lotusfoods.com.

Exotic Rice Dessert Crepes and Pancakes   (Serves 4 or more)

This recipe is similar to the dinner crepes. You'll be using the pancake as a base for the fruit. Note: Be especially careful handling the purple rice batter—it can stain!

For the pancake:
1 cup Lotus Foods' Forbidden Rice Flour*
2 tablespoons cornstarch, mixed with 3 tablespoons water
½ teaspoon honey
½ teaspoon sea salt
½ cup lite coconut milk
1 cup water, filtered or distilled
¼ cup walnut or pecan meal
3 tablespoons walnut or pecan pieces
2 whole eggs
1 teaspoon ground cinnamon (optional)

For the topping:
4 tablespoons frozen raspberries, defrosted
4 tablespoons frozen blueberries, defrosted
1 banana, thinly sliced
Greek yogurt (unsweetened) or just-made whipped cream

Mix all of the pancake ingredients together in a large bowl and whisk them by hand to blend. Heat a 6-inch nonstick frying pan over medium-high heat. When it's hot, pour some of the pancake batter into the center of the pan. You'll have to eyeball the right amount—the batter will start to solidify within seconds, so work quickly to spread the batter by tipping the pan. Cook the first side for 2 to 3 minutes, then carefully flip the pancake over, and cook the other side for another 2 minutes.

Transfer the pancakes to serving plates and spoon the fruit on top of the pancakes. Top them off with yogurt or whipped cream.

Alternatives: You can use Bhutanese Red Rice Flour, distributed by Lotus Foods. You can also use the pancake as a base for serving scrambled, fried, or poached eggs.

*This can be ordered at www.lotusfoods.com.

Hot and Cold Sauces and Marinades

These sauces and marinades add variety to sautéed chicken, fish, shrimp, and scallops. You can make these tasty sauces at home and freeze them in small amounts for future use. In general, I think they're tastier and more healthful than sauces you buy in a bottle. You may often have limited time, however, so it's all right to occasionally buy and use a bottled sauce from Trader Joe's or another specialty food store. Pesto sauces may be among the most reliable of store-bought sauces.

Traditional Pesto Sauce (Serves at least 4)

This pesto sauce works well with chicken, shrimp, scallops, and dense, strong-flavored fish, such as salmon. The recipe calls for making a large amount, dividing it into cubes, and freezing what you don't immediately use. That way, your initial investment in time will pay off with a quick, great-tasting sauce whenever you want one. You'll need a medium- to large-size food processor, two plastic ice-cube trays, and a ziplock plastic freezer bag. Most of your time will be spent preparing the ingredients. Once everything is in the food processor, the pesto will be ready in less than a minute.

4 cups basil leaves, stems removed (measure by packing the leaves tightly
　　into a 2-cup measuring cup)
4 garlic cloves, chopped
4 ounces pine nuts
½ teaspoon sea salt
1 cup Parmesan/Romano cheese blend, grated
1 cup extra-virgin Kalamata olive oil

The basil should be fresh, cleaned, and dry to the touch. Place the basil, garlic, and pine nuts in a 7-cup or larger food processor and grind them into a paste by repeatedly pressing the pulse button. Add the salt and cheese and grind everything until all the ingredients are thoroughly blended. Slowly add the olive oil while continuing to pulse and blend it with the ingredients. With a spatula, transfer the pesto to the cavities in the ice-cube trays and freeze them before the oil separates from the rest of the pesto.

Traditional Pesto Sauce *(continued)*

The next day, transfer the frozen pesto cubes to a ziplock freezer bag. When you want to use some of the pesto, defrost two to three cubes per pound of meat or shrimp. They'll defrost overnight in a small plastic container in the fridge or in a couple of hours on the countertop.

Easy Pesto Aioli

An aioli is a mayonnaise flavored with garlic. Most brands of store-bought mayo leave a lot to be desired in terms of ingredients and taste, but making your own mayo can be tricky. I use Spectrum Canola Mayonnaise, which I think is the highest quality and the tastiest mayo sold. (It's available at natural food stores.) You'll get the best results from this and other aioli recipes if you use Spectrum Canola Mayonnaise. This sauce works particularly well on sautéed or grilled salmon.

1 pesto cube, defrosted
1–2 tablespoons mayonnaise
juice from 1 lemon

With a fork, mix the pesto and mayonnaise. Squeeze the juice from one-quarter of a lemon, a little more if you would like a more liquid sauce. Use this aioli cold.

Mustard-Garlic Sauce

This sauce works well with Sautéed Shrimp (see page 97) or Sautéed Chicken Breast (see page 95).

4 garlic cloves, diced
1 teaspoon extra-virgin olive oil
1 pat butter
2 tablespoons Dijon mustard
1 tablespoon filtered or distilled water

Follow one of my sauté recipes to heat and soften the garlic in olive oil and butter. Add the shrimp or chicken. Meanwhile, mix the Dijon mustard and water in a small bowl and add this to the sautéing shrimp or chicken.

Saffron Sauce

This sauce works well with shrimp, scallops, or chicken breast slices.

½ teaspoon saffron
3 tablespoons filtered or distilled water
4 cloves garlic, diced
juice from ½ lemon

Working in or immediately above a small bowl, grind the saffron threads into a coarse powder with your thumb and index finger. Rinse your fingers so the saffron doesn't stain. Add the water and allow the saffron color to bleed into the water for about 15 minutes.

Follow my sauté recipes to soften the garlic and to start cooking the seafood or chicken. As it cooks, add the saffron-water mix. When the chicken or seafood is almost done, add the lemon juice.

Ginger Orange Sauce

This sauce works well with sautéed shrimp or scallops, or slices of chicken or pork.

¼ cup orange juice, fresh squeezed
½ tablespoon lime juice, fresh squeezed
1 teaspoon fresh ginger, peeled and finely grated
1 scallion, very finely sliced

In a small pan, mix all of the ingredients and bring them to a boil. Turn the heat down to low or medium and allow the liquid to reduce and thicken, until you have about ⅓ to ½ cup left.

Marinades

Marinades are essentially sauces that you immerse the food in for several hours before cooking. Typically, any leftover marinade is discarded because it may be contaminated by raw meat or seafood, although you can use some of it to cook with. Here are two simple marinades that work well with shrimp or chicken slices.

Lemon Garlic Rosemary Marinade

This marinade works well with seafood or chicken.

½ cup extra-virgin olive oil
4–6 garlic cloves, peeled and thinly sliced, chopped, or mashed (with the side
    of a knife)
4 sprigs fresh rosemary leaves, chopped
½ teaspoon sea salt
¼ teaspoon fresh ground black pepper
juice from 1 lemon

Mix all of the ingredients in a large glass bowl. Add the chicken, cover the bowl, and refrigerate it for 2 to 4 hours. If marinating seafood (such as shrimp, scallops, or white-colored fish), refrigerate it in the marinade for 20 to 30 minutes.

When you're ready to sauté, heat a small amount of olive oil in a non-stick frying pan over medium-high heat. Meanwhile, drain off the excess liquid from the bowl with the marinade. Add the marinated seafood or chicken to the pan and sauté until it's cooked. You may want to add a little more lemon juice while it's cooking.

Lemon Garlic Thyme Marinade

This marinade is perfect for seafood and chicken.

½ cup extra-virgin olive oil
4–6 garlic cloves, peeled and thinly sliced, chopped, or mashed (with the side
    of a knife)
4 sprigs fresh thyme leaves, chopped (if necessary)
½ teaspoon sea salt
¼ teaspoon fresh ground black pepper
juice from 1 lemon

Mix all of the ingredients in a large glass bowl. Add the chicken, cover the bowl, and refrigerate it for 2 to 4 hours. If marinating seafood (such as shrimp, scallops, or white-colored fish), refrigerate it in the marinade for 20 to 30 minutes.

When you're ready to sauté, heat a small amount of olive oil in a nonstick frying pan over medium-high heat. Meanwhile, drain off the excess liquid from the bowl with the marinade. Add the marinated seafood or chicken to the pan and sauté until it's cooked. You may want to add a little more lemon juice while it's cooking.

On the Grill

Grilled Fish and Veggies in Foil   (Serves 4)

This dish works well on a covered outdoor gas or charcoal grill, although you may have more control with a gas grill. It's great for patio or backyard dining with friends because you can prepare and refrigerate everything in advance. Serve the dish with cooked brown rice.

4 kale leaves or about 1 pound shredded cabbage (or cole slaw mix)
4 medium-size carrots, cleaned and thinly sliced
1 red bell pepper, sliced
1 yellow bell pepper, sliced
2 small- to medium-size zucchini squashes, sliced
1 small head of broccoli, cut into small florets
1 large red onion (or other sweet onion), thinly sliced
2 shallots, thinly sliced or chopped
extra-virgin olive oil
sea salt, to taste
fresh ground black pepper, to taste
4 fillets of a firm fish, such as salmon or tilapia
basil (dried or fresh), to taste
oregano (dried or fresh), to taste
2–3 cloves garlic, minced

Prepare the four servings on four sheets of aluminum foil, each about 1 square foot or so in size. (The shiny side of the foil should be against the food.) The bottom layer should be one or two leaves of kale or a bed of shredded cabbage. On top of this, arrange the other vegetables, with the harder ones toward the bottom and the softer ones toward the top, such as carrots, bell peppers, squash, broccoli, onions, and shallots. You can use different vegetables if you prefer. Drizzle about 1 teaspoon of olive oil on top of the veggies, along with salt and pepper. Next, place

Grilled Fish and Veggies in Foil *(continued)*

a fillet of salmon, tilapia, or another relatively firm fish on top of the veggies. Drizzle another teaspoon of olive oil on the fish and sprinkle on the basil, oregano, and garlic. Fold it up and secure the aluminum foil, making sure it is completely airtight and that the seam remains on top.

Preheat your grill to a medium setting and place each foil pack on the grill, leaving at least 1 inch between each one. Grill them for 12 to 15 minutes. The water in the vegetables and the seafood will steam-cook the food. When everything is done, transfer the foil packs to plates and carefully slice them open to serve.

Side Dishes for Dinner or Lunch

Steamed Vegetables   (Serves 2)

For this recipe, you'll need a 2-quart saucepan and an aluminum or plastic steamer that fits into the pot. These steamers typically have leaves that unfold like the petals of a flower.

½ head cauliflower, cut into florets
½ head broccoli, cut into florets
butter or coconut oil
salt, to taste

Place the steamer in the pot and add about 1 inch of water, so that it comes to the bottom of the steamer. Rinse the vegetables and place them in the steamer. Cover the pot, but leave it slightly ajar so that steam can escape. Heat it on high for 8 to 10 minutes, depending on whether you prefer your vegetables al dente or soft. Serve them with a small amount of butter or coconut oil and salt.

Optional: You can steam many other vegetables as well. Green beans and carrots will steam much faster, in 5 to 6 minutes.

Note: Always remove the cover after you steam vegetables. If you keep the cover on, the vegetables will continue steaming and will turn mushy.

Cauliflower and Almond Slices   (Serves 2–3)

1 head of cauliflower, cut into very small florets
1–2 tablespoons melted butter
1 tablespoon coconut oil
¼ cup almond slices

Steam the cauliflower for about 8 minutes. Transfer the cauliflower to a large bowl with a tight-fitting lid. Add the butter, coconut oil, and almond slices; cover the bowl and shake it to mix the ingredients.

Optional: While steaming the cauliflower, toast the almonds in a hot but dry frying pan.

Sautéed Vegetables   (Serves 2)

1 tablespoon extra-virgin olive oil
1 pat butter
½ cup fresh mushrooms, sliced
¼ cup red bell peppers, diced
¼ cup scallions or red onions, diced
½ teaspoon dried basil
1 teaspoon dried oregano
1 cup baby spinach leaves, stems removed
3 tablespoons Romano cheese, shredded

Heat a large frying pan over medium-high heat. Add the olive oil and butter. When the butter melts and sizzles, add the mushrooms, peppers, and onions. Mix them with a heat-resistant spatula. Add the basil and oregano and stir everything throughout. When the vegetables start to soften, add the spinach leaves and mix them so that the heat wilts them slightly. Add the Romano cheese, allow it to melt a little, and serve.

Broiled Asparagus   (Serves 3)

12 ounces fresh asparagus spears
extra-virgin olive oil
¼ red onion, thinly sliced
1 tablespoon fresh sage, chopped

Cut off the woody 1-inch bottoms of the asparagus stems. Then use a vegetable peeler to remove the peel along the lower parts of the stems. Spread a thin layer of olive oil on a baking sheet and lay the asparagus spears on it. Arrange the onion slices on top of the asparagus. Drizzle them with olive oil and sprinkle them with sage. Broil them for 3 to 5 minutes with the asparagus about 3 inches from the heating element. Use tongs to flip the asparagus over and bake for another 2 to 3 minutes. The asparagus is done when the tips start to have a seared, crunchy look.

Rosemary Carrots   (Serves 3)

8 ounces baby carrots or large carrots, cut into ¼-inch-thick circles
extra-virgin olive oil
2 teaspoons fresh or dried rosemary leaves, chopped
garlic powder

Clean and peel the carrots as necessary and place them in a microwave-safe bowl. Drizzle the olive oil over the carrots and sprinkle the rosemary leaves and garlic powder over them. Microwave the carrots at medium-high power for 5 to 10 minutes. (Cooking times vary with different types of microwave ovens.) The carrots will cook for another 1 or 2 minutes after being heated.

Short- or Long-Grain Brown Rice

Once you've had a flavorful colored rice, you'll probably find most types of white rice bland and boring. Limit your quantities if you are overweight or have glucose-tolerance problems.

1 cup rice
1 cup organic, free-range chicken or vegetable broth (such as Pacific brand)
1 cup filtered water

Rinse the rice in a strainer and transfer it to a 1- or 2-quart saucepan. Add the broth and water and cover the saucepan with the top slightly ajar. Bring it to a boil over high heat, about 5 minutes. Reduce the heat to low and allow the rice to cook for 40 to 45 minutes. (The time will vary by a few minutes, depending on your stove and the altitude.)

Brown Jasmine Rice   (Serves 4)

Jasmine rice is one of the most aromatic of all rices. If friends drop by while I'm cooking it, their mouths always water and they wonder what I'm cooking up in the kitchen.

1 cup jasmine rice
1 cup organic, free-range chicken broth (such as Pacific brand)
1 cup filtered water

Rinse the rice in a strainer and transfer it to a 1- or 2-quart saucepan. Add the broth and water. Bring it to a boil over high heat, about 5 minutes. Cover the saucepan tightly and reduce the heat to a simmer for 35 to 40 minutes. Turn off the heat and let the rice sit for 5 to 10 minutes. Fluff up the rice with a fork and serve.

Purple Rice   (Serves 4)

1 cup Lotus Foods' Forbidden Rice*
1 cup organic, free-range chicken broth (such as Pacific brand)
¾ cup filtered water

Rinse the rice in a strainer and transfer it to a 1- or 2-quart saucepan. Add the broth and water. Bring it to a boil over high heat, about 5 minutes. Cover the saucepan tightly and reduce the heat to a simmer for about 30 minutes. Fluff up the rice with a fork and serve.

*This can be ordered at www.lotusfoods.com.

Wild Rice   (Serves 4)

Wild rice is actually a grass, not a rice. It has a full-bodied flavor.

1 cup wild rice
1 cup high-quality chicken or vegetable broth (such as Pacific brand)
2 cups water
2 stalks celery, diced
4 ounces water chestnuts, diced
2–3 tablespoons organic raisins

Rinse the rice in a strainer and transfer it to a 2-quart saucepan. Add the broth and water. Bring it to a boil over high heat, about 5 minutes. Cover the saucepan tightly and reduce the heat to a simmer. After 20 minutes, add the celery, water chestnuts, and raisins to the rice and stir. The rice should cook fully in 40 to 50 minutes. Fluff it with a fork and drain off any excess water. The rice should be al dente; do not overcook it.

Very Fast Lunches

On-the-Run Blood Sugar Stabilizer   (Serves 1)

How often do you skip lunch because you're too busy to eat? Here's a quick solution if you work in a place where you can refrigerate these simple ingredients. If you work from a car or a truck, this lunch is as close as the deli counter at a supermarket—or you can store the cheese and meat in a cooler.

3 slices deli cheese, such as light Swiss
3 slices deli turkey, chicken, beef, or ham
mustard

On a plate or a paper towel, lay out two or three slices of cheese. On top of each one, place a slice of turkey, chicken, beef, or ham. Squeeze a little mustard on top of the meat, then fold the cheese and meat between your fingers. *Note*: I recommend *against* using salami, any other type of sausage meat, or any prepackaged meat.

Quick-and-Easy Roll-Up   (Serves 1)

You can prepare this simple lunch the night before. I often make a couple of these roll-ups when I have to fly or drive on business and I know there won't be many healthy food options along the way.

1 whole wheat, low-carb tortilla
2 slices cheese, such as light Swiss
1 slice deli turkey, chicken, beef, or ham
mustard or canola mayonnaise
1–2 pickled asparagus spears*
tomato, 2 thin slices

Lay a sheet of aluminum foil on your counter and put the tortilla on top of it. Place the cheese and meat on the tortilla and spread them with mustard or mayonnaise (or both). Add the asparagus spears and the tomato slices. Carefully roll the tortilla, then wrap the foil around it. Twist the bottom and top of the foil. When you're ready to eat the roll-up, start peeling away the foil from one side.

    Alternatives: You can use other fillings, such as avocado or cucumber.

Cold Plate Lunch   (Serves 1)

Europeans are masters at creating tasty cold plate lunches. I recommend breaking with tradition by avoiding the bread and instead enjoying a few Nut-Thins brand crackers (made mostly with nuts, not wheat), which are available at natural food markets.

2–3 slices cheese
2–3 slices deli turkey, chicken, beef, or ham
marinated vegetables, such as mushrooms, asparagus, carrots, or baby corn
cucumber, tomato, avocado, or roasted red pepper, sliced
mustard, canola mayonnaise, or horseradish
stuffed grape leaves
Nut-Thins brand crackers†

*From Point Reyes Preserves—see the appendix for details.
†These can be ordered at www.bluediamond.com.

Cold Plate Lunch *(continued)*

Simply assemble the ingredients on a dinner plate.

Optional: You can dip the crackers in hummus, a chickpea dip that's sold in most supermarkets.

Avocado and Roasted Bell Peppers   (Serves 1)

This is a quick, healthy snack that keeps me going when I can't take a break for a full lunch at the normal hour.

1 avocado, ripe but firm
2–3 tablespoons roasted red bell pepper (sold in jars), diced
flavorful salad dressing

Slice the avocado in half, beginning where the stem was. Remove the pit. Spoon the diced red pepper into the depressions where the pit had been. Drizzle some dressing over the red pepper. Eat it with a small spoon, scraping the avocado from the skin. Alternatively, you can remove the avocado from the skin, slice it in a bowl or on a plate, and spread the diced red peppers and dressing over the avocado.

My favorite dressing for this is Stonewall Kitchen's Roasted Garlic, but you can experiment with other healthy creamy dressings from Stonewall Kitchen or Annie's Naturals.

Lunches

Turkey Tacos   (Serves 2–4)

I try to avoid using prepackaged sauces and blends of seasonings, but the McCormick brand Taco Seasoning is about the best for a fast and incredibly easy meal.

1–1½ pounds ground turkey (or beef)
1 packet McCormick Taco Seasoning
¾ cup water
low-carb whole wheat or corn tortillas

Follow the package directions—break the ground turkey into small pieces and brown them in a large nonstick frying pan over medium heat. Continue to break up the turkey pieces with a spatula until they are small. Drain the fat. Sprinkle in the seasoning and water; mix everything thoroughly. Continue cooking the turkey at a simmer until most of the water is gone. Spoon the ground turkey into low-carb whole wheat or corn tortillas.

Optional: Top the tacos with chopped lettuce, diced tomatoes, shredded cheese, sour cream, or guacamole.

Note: Save some of the cooked Turkey Taco meat in a sealed container in the fridge. You can use it in my Mexican-Style Omelet (see page 128), Breakfast Huevos (see page 129), and Breakfast Burrito (see page 129) recipes.

Turkey Taco Salad   (Serves 2–4)

1–1½ pounds ground turkey (or beef)
1 packet McCormick Taco Seasoning
refried beans, shredded cheese, diced scallions, shredded lettuce, diced
    tomatoes, guacamole, sour cream (optional)

Prepare the ground turkey as you did for the Turkey Tacos (above), or use leftover cooked and seasoned meat. On a plate, spread about 1 cup of cooked Turkey Taco meat in a small circle. Layer whichever toppings you would like: refried beans, shredded cheese, diced scallions, shredded lettuce, diced tomatoes, guacamole, or sour cream.

Guacamole   (Serves 2–3)

2 ripe avocados
2–3 tablespoons red, yellow, and orange bell peppers, finely diced
1–2 tablespoons shallots (about 1 medium head), finely diced
3–4 tablespoons cilantro (leaves from several sprigs), chopped
½ teaspoon garlic powder
¼ teaspoon ground coriander
¼ teaspoon ground (dried) red pepper

Guacamole *(continued)*

juice from 1 lime
Terrapin Ridge Yellow Pepper Squeeze* (optional)
½ teaspoon jalapeño pepper, finely minced (optional)

Place the avocado fruit in a glass bowl (discard the skin and seed) and mash it with a fork. Add all of the other ingredients, including the Yellow Pepper Squeeze and jalapeño, if using. Continue to mash and mix until you develop a nice consistency, not too dry and not too wet. Add more cilantro and lime juice if you wish. Refrigerate, but plan to use it within 1 hour. Remix the guacamole immediately before use.

Quesadillas   (Serves 1)

pat of butter
2 small low-carb whole-wheat tortillas
Turkey Taco meat, cooked (see Turkey Tacos recipe on page 118)
shredded cheese, white or yellow
scallions or chives, finely chopped
sour cream or guacamole

Melt the butter in a 12-inch nonstick frying pan over medium heat. Place one tortilla in the pan, and after about 30 seconds, add a little meat and spread the cheese. Add the scallions or chives, then place the other tortilla on top. With a large spatula, carefully flip the quesadilla and continue to fry it for about 1 minute. Transfer the quesadilla to a plate and serve it with guacamole or sour cream.

Salads for Lunch and Dinner

Salads are among the healthiest meals you can make, and my Quick-and-Easy Chicken Caesar Salad provides both high-quality protein and tasty veggies.

*This can be ordered at www.terrapinridge.com.

When ordering salad in a restaurant, you have to watch out for two things: croutons and the dressing. Croutons are nothing more than empty carb calories; ask your waiter to leave them off. While better restaurants make their own salad dressings, most chain and fast-food restaurants rely on prepackaged salad dressings, which usually are made from soybean oil, "partially hydrogenated vegetable oil," and some type of sugar. You don't want any of these ingredients. If a nutritionally awful salad dressing is what you're faced with, ask for a little olive oil and vinegar mixed together. Balsamic, red wine, and apple cider vinegars are fine.

Quick-and-Easy Chicken Caesar Salad   (Serves 1)

Romaine lettuce hearts are nutritious, have a wonderful flavor, and can easily stay for two weeks in the refrigerator if they are well sealed.

romaine hearts
pan-fried chicken breast
1–3 tablespoons Parmesan or Romano cheese, shredded or flaked
bottled dressing, such as Annie's Naturals Caesar Dressing

Remove any wilted or brown leaves from the romaine. Lay the romaine hearts on a cutting board, thinly slice them across the top, and work your way down to the base. Discard the pulpy base. Rinse the cut leaves in a colander, then pat them dry with paper towels. Transfer the lettuce to a large bowl. Next, thinly slice part or all of a cooked and cooled chicken breast and add it to the salad bowl. (See my recipe for Sautéed Chicken Breast on page 95.) Sprinkle on Parmesan or Romano cheese, and toss the salad with a high-quality Caesar dressing, such as Annie's Naturals Caesar Dressing (available at health food stores).

Note: I find that shredded or flaked Parmesan or Romano cheese tastes better than grated. You can buy it in these forms or shred it yourself with a large-holed grater.

Shrimp and Cucumber Salad   (Serves 1–2)

1 cup salad shrimp
1 cup cucumbers, preferably Persian or English style, thinly sliced
3 very thin slices red onion, rings separated
½ teaspoon dried basil
½ teaspoon dried oregano
1 tablespoon extra-virgin olive oil
1–2 tablespoons balsamic vinegar
juice from 1 lemon
sea salt, to taste
fresh ground black pepper, to taste
romaine lettuce, shredded or finely sliced

Mix the shrimp, cucumbers, and red onion together in a bowl. Add the basil and oregano, followed by the olive oil and balsamic vinegar. Squeeze lemon juice onto the salad. Add salt and pepper. Refrigerate the salad for several hours before eating it. Serve the salad on a bed of shredded or finely sliced romaine lettuce.

   Alternative: Skip the basil, oregano, olive oil, and vinegar.

Curried Chicken Salad   (Serves 2–4)

1 pound cooked chicken breasts (see Sautéed Chicken Breast recipe on
   page 95)
½ cup celery, chopped
¼ cup flavorful apple, such as Gala variety, diced
2 tablespoons raisins, preferably organically grown
⅛ to ¼ cup pecans, chopped
½ cup or so high-quality mayonnaise (such as Spectrum Canola Mayonnaise)
½ to 1 teaspoon curry powder
½ to 1 teaspoon apple cider vinegar
⅛ teaspoon ground red pepper
fresh ground black pepper, to taste
salt, to taste

Dice the chicken and place it in a large mixing bowl. Add the celery, apple, raisins, and pecans and mix them together using a large spoon.

Add about ½ cup of mayonnaise, but adjust the amount according to whether you like it creamy or relatively dry. Likewise, adjust the amount of curry powder, vinegar, and red pepper to your taste, and season the salad with a small amount of fresh ground black pepper and salt.

Tossed Salad   (Serves 2)

3 cups romaine lettuce, chopped, or baby spinach leaves, or arugula
6–10 cherry tomatoes
1 small cucumber, sliced
3 tablespoons red bell pepper, diced
2 tablespoons scallions, chopped
3 tablespoons unsalted cashews or pecans
1 avocado, sliced
2 slices deli turkey or chicken, diced
2 tablespoons Romano cheese, shredded
hearts of palm, marinated artichoke hearts (optional)

In a large bowl, toss together all of the ingredients with a pair of salad tongs or two large forks. You can use some or all of the listed ingredients, depending on your taste. Add some salad dressing (see upcoming recipes) and toss it again to lightly coat the vegetables.

Salad Dressings

These salad dressings are easy to prepare and will stay fresh for several days in the refrigerator. Vary your dressings to keep your salads from getting boring.

Simple Oil and Vinegar Dressing

When making oil and vinegar dressing, you can vary the relative proportions of olive oil and vinegar from 1:1 to 1:3. Studies have found that 2 tablespoons of vinegar have an appetite-reducing effect and also improve both blood sugar and insulin levels, so I tend to use a little more vinegar.

Simple Oil and Vinegar Dressing *(continued)*

¼ cup extra-virgin olive oil
¼ to ⅜ cup balsamic vinegar
½ to 1 teaspoon dried basil
½ to 1 teaspoon dried oregano
juice from a quarter wedge of lemon (optional)

Mix together the ingredients and stir or shake them. You can use the dressing immediately or refrigerate it for later use. Always shake the dressing before using it because the ingredients might settle or separate.

Apple Cider Vinaigrette Dressing

¼ cup extra-virgin olive oil
¼ to ½ cup apple cider vinegar
½–2 teaspoons Dijon mustard

Mix the olive oil and vinegar and stir. Add a small amount of the mustard, which will thicken the dressing a little. You can add more if you'd like a thicker dressing. Use the dressing immediately or refrigerate it. The ingredients may separate, so always shake the dressing before using it.

Raspberry Vinaigrette

2 tablespoons raspberry balsamic vinaigrette
6 tablespoons extra-virgin olive oil
2 teaspoons fresh lemon juice
2 teaspoons shallot, minced
salt and pepper, to taste

Combine the ingredients and whisk or stir vigorously. You can store what you don't use in a sealed container in the refrigerator for about a week.

Cherry Vinaigrette

2 tablespoons cherry balsamic vinaigrette
6 tablespoons extra-virgin olive oil
2 teaspoons fresh lemon juice
2 teaspoons shallot, minced
salt and pepper, to taste

Combine the ingredients and whisk or stir vigorously. You can store what you don't use in a sealed container in the refrigerator for about a week.

Citrus-Lime Dressing

½ cup extra-virgin olive oil
2 teaspoons vinegar, such as balsamic, red wine, or apple cider
2 tablespoons lemon juice, freshly squeezed
½ cup orange juice, freshly squeezed

Mix the ingredients, adjusting the amounts to suit your taste.

Optional: Add six to eight finely minced cilantro leaves, then blend all the ingredients in a blender.

Lime-Cilantro Vinaigrette

½ cup fresh lime juice
½ cup white wine, champagne, or sherry vinegar
cilantro leaves from one bunch, chopped, with stems removed
¼ cup honey
1 tablespoon fresh garlic, chopped
2 tablespoons coarse-grain Dijon mustard
1½–2 cups extra-virgin olive oil

Combine the ingredients in a blender or a food processor. Puree them until the dressing is smooth. You can tweak the taste and reduce the thickness by adding a little more lime juice or white wine.

Breakfast

Scrambled Egg   (Serves 1)

This is a quick, simple breakfast that nearly anyone can find time to prepare.

½ teaspoon extra-virgin olive oil or 1 pat butter
1 large egg
1 teaspoon or so Romano or Parmesan cheese, shredded

Heat a small nonstick frying pan over medium-high heat. Add the olive oil or butter. Meanwhile, beat 1 large egg in a small bowl and pour it into the pan. Allow it to cook until set for about 20 seconds, then move it around in the pan with a heat-resistant spatula. Sprinkle on the cheese and serve the egg with a small amount of fresh fruit on the side.

Hard-Boiled Eggs   (Serves 1–2)

2–4 large eggs (still in the shell)
water

Place the eggs in a 1-quart saucepan. Add enough water to cover the eggs and bring to a boil over high heat. Remove the pot from the burner, cover it, and allow the eggs to cook in the hot water for 25 minutes. Rinse the eggs in cool water, pat dry, and refrigerate them until you use them over the next several days.

Alternatives: To serve, remove the shell and slice the egg in half lengthwise. Sprinkle on a little sea salt and fresh ground black pepper or sea salt and paprika. Or, dip the egg in a small amount of Traditional Pesto Sauce (see page 107), Easy Pesto Aioli (see page 108), or Mustard-Garlic Sauce (see page 108).

Real Simple Omelet   (Serves 1)

1 teaspoon olive oil or 1 pat butter
2–3 eggs, beaten
1 tablespoon Romano, Parmesan, or Double Gloucester cheese, shredded

Heat a small nonstick frying pan over medium-high heat. Add the olive oil or butter. Pour the eggs into the pan and allow them to cook until set, about 1 minute. Tip the pan and lift one side of the omelet with a spatula to let the uncooked egg flow underneath. Reduce the heat to medium. Either let the omelet continue cooking until the egg becomes mostly firm, or flip the omelet over to cook the other side for about 30 seconds. Whichever way you choose, when the omelet is almost cooked, sprinkle the cheese on one side and fold over the omelet.

Fruity Omelet   (Serves 1)

You can buy bags of frozen blueberries and raspberries at most grocers, natural food stores, and Trader Joe's. They work better than fresh for this recipe because the frozen berries release some of their water as they defrost, and the water forms a light sauce.

1 tablespoon frozen blueberries, defrosted
1 tablespoon frozen raspberries, defrosted
1 teaspoon olive oil
1 pat butter
2–3 eggs

The night before, place a small amount of frozen blueberries and raspberries in a small plastic container and keep it in the fridge to thaw out. To make the omelet, heat a small nonstick frying pan over medium heat, then add the olive oil and melt the butter. Beat the eggs and pour them into the pan. Allow the eggs to cook until they're set, probably a couple of minutes. When the eggs are firm enough, flip the omelet. Place the berries on one side of the omelet, fold over the other side, and serve.

Scrambled Eggs and Sautéed Veggies   (Serves 2)

1 tablespoon extra-virgin olive oil
1 pat butter
½ cup fresh mushrooms, sliced
¼ cup red bell pepper, chopped or diced
¼ cup scallions or red onion, chopped or diced
⅛ cup cooked brown rice
½ cup spinach leaves, stems removed
4 eggs, beaten
2 tablespoons Romano cheese, shredded

Scrambled Eggs and Sautéed Vegetables *(continued)*

Heat a wok over medium-high heat. Add the oil and butter. When the butter melts and is hot, add the mushrooms, red pepper, and onion and mix them together. Sauté the vegetables to your preference, al dente or soft. Add the rice and mix everything. Add the spinach and stir it with the other vegetables. Move the vegetables to one side and add the egg, allowing it to cook until set for about 1 minute. Then mix all of the ingredients together, except the cheese. When the eggs are just about cooked—that is, when the egg whites are solid—turn off the heat, add the cheese, and mix.

Save the leftovers by immediately placing them in a bowl, covering it, and refrigerating. You can reheat them in the microwave within a day or two.

Tip: I often dice the red peppers and scallions ahead of time and keep them refrigerated in a sealed plastic container so they're ready to use when I need them.

Mexican-Style Omelet   (Serves 1)

1 pat butter or 1 teaspoon macadamia nut oil
2 or 3 eggs
Turkey Taco meat, cooked (see Turkey Tacos on page 118)
2 tablespoons shredded cheese, white or yellow
chives, chopped

Heat a nonstick frying pan over medium-high heat, then add the butter or macadamia nut oil. Beat the eggs and pour them into the pan. Allow the eggs to cook until they're set, 1 to 2 minutes, flip the omelet, then add the Turkey Taco meat, shredded cheese, and chives on one side. Fold the other half of the omelet over it.

Breakfast Huevos   (Serves 1)

1 pat butter or 1 teaspoon macadamia nut oil
2 eggs
Turkey Taco meat, cooked (see Turkey Tacos on page 118)

Heat a nonstick frying pan over medium-high heat, then add the butter or macadamia nut oil. Beat the eggs and pour them into the pan. Allow the eggs to cook until set, 1 to 2 minutes, then add a small amount of the Turkey Taco meat. Stir everything with a spatula until the eggs are scrambled and cooked.

Note: The scrambled eggs and Turkey Taco meat can be safely stored in the refrigerator for 2 days and can be reused to make a Breakfast Burrito (see the next recipe). To store, place the cooked eggs and Turkey Taco meat in a sealed container and refrigerate it immediately. Reheat it in the microwave.

Breakfast Burrito   (Serves 1)

macadamia nut oil or extra-virgin olive oil
1 egg
Turkey Taco meat, cooked (see Turkey Tacos on page 118)
1 tablespoon cheese, shredded
1 whole wheat, low-carb tortilla

Heat a nonstick frying pan over medium-high heat, then add a little macadamia nut oil or olive oil. Pour in the egg and scramble it with a spatula. As the egg starts to firm, add a small amount of the Turkey Taco meat. Meanwhile, heat the tortilla at medium in the microwave for 10 seconds. Spread the scrambled eggs on one side of the tortilla, then begin rolling it from that side.

Fruit Salad   (Serves 2–4)

Fruit salads are a great side dish with breakfast eggs, or they can be eaten as an after-dinner dessert. You can make this fruit salad with as few ingredients as you wish or as many, using whatever happens to be in season. The yogurt helps to preserve the fruit salad for at least two days in the fridge.

1 banana, sliced
1 apple, cut into chunks
1 kiwifruit, cut into chunks
1 cup cantaloupe, cut into chunks
1 heavy tablespoon pomegranate seeds
¼ cup frozen raspberries, defrosted
¼ cup frozen blueberries, defrosted
2 tablespoons pecan or walnut pieces
yogurt, preferably sugar- and fat-free Fage brand of Greek yogurt
½–1 teaspoon ground cinnamon

Mix the fruit and nuts together with a spoon, add the yogurt, then the cinnamon. You can vary the ingredients with whatever happens to be in season.

Sample Two-Week Meal Plan

This menu plan is intended as a list of meal options, not a rigid diet plan. You can certainly switch meals around and make extensive use of leftovers to save time in preparing meals. For example, many dinner leftovers work well when chopped and mixed with scrambled eggs. It's also easy to take leftovers to work and reheat them in a microwave oven—high-quality meals lead to tasty leftovers. An asterisk (*) indicates that the recipe is in this book. Other recipes can easily be found in cookbooks and on the Internet.

Sunday (Day 1)

Breakfast	Scrambled Egg with side of Fresh Fruit*
Lunch	Turkey Tacos* with Guacamole*
Dinner	Braised Beef Brisket*

Monday (Day 2)

Breakfast	Hard-Boiled Eggs* with sea salt and paprika
Lunch	Turkey Taco Salad*
Dinner	Seared Ahi Tuna*

Tuesday (Day 3)

Breakfast	Hard-Boiled Eggs with Pesto Aioli*
Lunch	Cold Plate Lunch (deli meats and cheeses, vegetables)*
Dinner	Sautéed Chicken Breast*

Wednesday (Day 4)

Breakfast	Mexican-Style Omelet*
Lunch	Deli Roll-Ups (with meat and cheese)*
Dinner	Sautéed Shrimp*

Thursday (Day 5)

Breakfast	Real Simple Omelet*
Lunch	Chicken Caesar Salad*
Dinner	Pan-Fried Salmon with Pesto*

Friday (Day 6)

Breakfast	Scrambled Egg with Purple Rice Pancake*
Lunch	Shrimp and Cucumber Salad*
Dinner	Baked Cornish hen

Saturday (Day 7)

Breakfast	Fruity Omelet*
Lunch	Shrimp fajitas
Dinner	Grilled Fish and Vegetables*

Sunday (Day 8)

Breakfast	Scrambled Eggs and Sautéed Vegetables*
Lunch	Hamburger with steamed vegetables
Dinner	Roast Chicken*

Monday (Day 9)

Breakfast   Breakfast Burrito*

Lunch   Greek Salad*

Dinner   Exotic Red Rice Crepes* with leftover chicken and gravy

Tuesday (Day 10)

Breakfast   Omelet with pieces of cooked fish

Lunch   Chicken Rice Soup*

Dinner   Trout almondine

Wednesday (Day 11)

Breakfast   Eggs Florentine without the muffin

Lunch   Tuna salad

Dinner   Pan-Fried Dumplings*

Thursday (Day 12)

Breakfast   Real Simple Omelet*

Lunch   Curried Chicken Salad,* with small tossed green salad

Dinner   Pan-fried fillet of sole

Friday (Day 13)

Breakfast   Scrambled Egg*

Lunch   Lamb burger with steamed vegetables

Dinner   Baked turkey breast

Saturday (Day 14)

Breakfast   Omelet with chicken pieces and avocado slices

Lunch   Turkey salad, with a small tossed green salad

Dinner   Chicken Piccata* with rice and vegetables

6

The Third Step:
Be More Active

I used to be a classic couch potato. While I've always enjoyed long walks and an occasional hike, my work as a writer has been sedentary, and I spent most evenings reading books or watching television. Then, at fifty-three, I was introduced to cycling by a friend. At first, it felt like torture. After I struggled to the top of my first hill, my heart was pounding and my lungs were straining.

I've since come to enjoy my brisk bike rides, zipping along the snaking paths of a nearby river park for fourteen to twenty miles several mornings a week. I discovered that cycling could clear my head of stress, and it's been great for my physical health as well. My energy levels are higher, and I've gained more muscle. Cycling has also reduced my cholesterol and triglyceride levels and improved my glucose tolerance—that is, resistance to diabetes. If I can learn to be more physically active, so can you. It's easier than you think.

I've long known that exercise is important for health, but I've also understood how nonathletes usually dread the E word. Hearing the word *exercise* can send couch potatoes running to the nearest sofa with thoughts of fatigue, embarrassment, and an already overloaded schedule.

Instead, I've learned to recommend *physical activity*. Physical activity doesn't have to be structured, such as going to a gym every day. Nor does it have to be painful, like the jogger who looks like he's about to collapse. It doesn't have to be competitive. And it doesn't have to feel like exercise. Physical activity can and should be fun, just the way it was when we were kids.

Physical Activity and Mood

We all know that physical activity is good for the heart and reduces cholesterol levels, but it's also great for your mood. Researchers have known since at least the 1970s that regular physical activity can significantly reduce symptoms of depression, with benefits comparable to the best antidepressant medications. Physical activity can also reduce anxiety, as well as improve overall mood and outlook on life.

Why would physical activity have such a positive influence on mood? There are several reasons, some of which are chemical and others psychological (but that, in turn, improve brain chemistry). They're all good examples of the body-mind connection.

- Physical activity reduces stress-related neurotransmitters, including cortisol and epinephrine (adrenaline).

- Physical activity increases the production of endorphins, brain chemicals that enhance mood.

- Physical activity improves how your body uses insulin and glucose, which lessens mood swings.

- Physical activity increases muscle, which is the best type of tissue for burning glucose and fat.

- Physical activity speeds up the metabolic rate—that is, the speed of biochemical reactions in cells. These reactions stimulate the production of necessary chemicals throughout the body and the removal of waste products from cells.

- Physical activity keeps you slimmer, and thinner people are less prone than overweight people to depression and anxiety.

- Physical activity can promote feelings of self-esteem and self-confidence, as well as distract you from mood problems.

- Physical activities with other people often lead to positive social feedback and reinforcement.

It almost doesn't matter what type of physical activity you engage in or how intense it is, as long as it's regular—even for as little as ten minutes—each day or several times a week.

Of course, the more physical activity you engage in, the greater the benefits. That was the finding of a study by Andrea L. Dunn, Ph.D., of the Cooper Institute in Golden, Colorado. Like taking more of a vitamin (within reason, of course), larger amounts of physical activity have a more dramatic effect on mood compared with less strenuous activities. Dunn studied eighty young and middle-aged adults with mild to serious depression. She found that moderate (three days a week) physical activity for twelve weeks reduced symptoms of depression by 30 percent; however, more intense (five days a week) aerobic exercise cut symptoms of depression by almost half!

Researchers have consistently found that vigorous physical activity alleviates feelings of depression and improves mood, regardless of a person's age. For example, studies have shown powerful mood-enhancing benefits for teenagers, young adults, middle-aged adults, and seniors. Again, the benefits are comparable to the best medications—and without side effects.

Similarly, physical activity reduces anxiety levels. In one study of forty-three anxiety patients, researchers reported that regular aerobic exercise improved heart function, glucose metabolism, and mood. Another study found that even small amounts of routine daily physical activity—not exercise, per se—led to less anxiety and better moods.

How to Make Your First Move

Stage 1: Get Started

I'll be the first to admit that it's not easy to start a regular regimen of physical activity and, once started, not to be discouraged by how tired and sore you feel. The payoff of actually feeling better usually takes several weeks, and that can seem like an eternity. Try the following steps, and you might find the first few weeks of an exercise program more tolerable.

- *Figure out what you really want to accomplish.* Do you want to reduce feelings of depression or anxiety? Lessen your long-term risk of diabetes or heart disease? Improve your energy levels? Some types of activities will be better than others for achieving specific objectives.

- *Start slow and easy.* If you're out of shape, begin exercising slowly but regularly. For example, walking is a great way to start. You can do it early in the morning, during lunch, or after work and dinner. If you're really out of shape—you know whether you are or aren't—start with a ten-minute daily walk. As soon as you're able to, perhaps after a week or two, increase it to fifteen minutes, then twenty, and then thirty minutes. In addition to walking longer distances, try picking up your pace a little. Walking will lower blood sugar levels, improve glucose tolerance, and produce modest cardiovascular benefits.

- *Bring a friend.* We're social creatures, so it might be more fun to exercise with a significant other, a coworker, or a neighbor. Talking with another person helps to get your mind off the activity. Dancing

Quick Tip

Hand Weights: Simple and Easy

You don't have to go to a gym to start building your arm and upper body muscles. If you've been sedentary, buy two five-pound (or adjustable) hand weights at a sporting goods store and work with them at home.

Exercise #1. Sit in a firm chair, with your back straight and your feet flat on the ground. You should have one hand weight in each hand, and your arms should be along your sides, with the weights at about hip level. Raise both hand weights so that they almost touch your shoulders; your palms should face your head. Exhale while lifting the weights. Inhale as you bring the weights back to a resting position next to your hips. Take one breath, then repeat. Do eight reps (repetitions) and rest for a minute or two. Do another eight reps, but this time alternate between using your left and right hands. Repeat.

Exercise #2. Sit in a firm chair, with your back straight and your feet flat on the ground, one hand weight in each hand. Raise the weights to your shoulder, with the palms of your hands facing forward. This is your starting position. Exhale as you lift the weights so that your arms are straight up. Inhale as you go back to your starting position. Take one breath, then repeat. Do eight reps, rest for a minute or two, and do another eight reps. Repeat.

is a great physical activity for couples if you have a partner who also enjoys it.

- *Find a nice location.* It might be your own neighborhood, downtown, or a park. If you're concerned about safety, consider walking in an indoor shopping mall. Many of them allow walkers to come in to walk before the stores open.

Stage 2: Build on What You've Accomplished

After increasing your stamina, continue to build on what you've accomplished.

- *Which exercises appeal to you?* Increasing your physical activity is often a series of stepping-stones. Besides walking, which exercises do you imagine being good at? Tennis demands good hand-eye coordination, which you can learn. Cycling requires some sense of balance. Some exercises can be either solo or group activities. Think about whether you want to interact with another person while exercising, or whether you'd rather enjoy a little solitude.

- *Which exercises seem best suited to you?* Different people are genetically better suited to certain types of exercises. Michelle Lovitt and John Speraw, the authors of *Exercise for Your Muscle Type*, explain that people tend to have either mostly slow-twitch or fast-twitch muscle fibers. Your predominant type of muscle fiber will determine which exercises you're likely to be most suited for.

  Slow-twitch muscles are best for steady, low-force aerobic activities, including aerobic dance, cycling, hiking, jogging, snow shoeing, stair climbing, swimming, and walking. In contrast, fast-twitch muscles are better for short bursts of energy, such as those required for baseball, basketball, golf, handball, martial arts, skiing, sprinting, tennis, weight lifting, and yoga.

Important Considerations while Exercising

- *Stay hydrated.* Physical activity should make you sweat, and that means you need to stay hydrated. Take regular breaks to drink water. If you're going to exercise nonstop for thirty minutes or more, bring water and an energy bar with you. (I consider the

Larabar and the Buzzbar brands to be the tastiest and most health-ful energy bars on the market.)

- *Work with a mentor*. Learn from people with more experience so that you train correctly and don't injure yourself. This doesn't mean you have to hire a personal trainer or join a gym. Your mentor could just be a good friend who has been exercising longer than you.

- *Remember to stretch*. Stretching limbers up your back and muscles before and after exercising. *A simple stretch*: Lie on your back on the floor with your legs straight. Lift one knee to your chest for ten seconds, straighten the leg, and repeat with your other knee. Next, stand with your feet a few inches apart. Slowly bend forward and bend your knees slightly, allowing your fingertips to touch your feet or ankles for five seconds.

- *Carb and protein intake*. Many athletes and weekend warriors believe that carbohydrate loading increases the amount of sugar (glycogen) stored in your liver, but carb loading can actually play havoc with blood sugar and insulin levels, making you feel more tired than energized, according to Loren Cordain, Ph.D., of Colorado State University, Fort Collins. Cordain, the author of *The Paleo Diet*, warns against carb loading. Instead, he suggests that people consume a mix of healthy carbs and protein (think fruit and turkey slices, as an example) during the postexercise recovery period, when the body starts to repair muscle damage. Muscle, after all, is made of protein.

In the next chapter, I describe ways that you can create more time and have less stress and greater balance in your life. Thus, you will be less dependent on supplements or medications to maintain healthy moods and behavior.

7

The Fourth Step:
Begin Changing Your
Life Habits

One thing that causes the greatest stress in our lives is having too much to do and too little time to do it in.

Contemporary life places tremendous demands on our time, and we rarely feel as if we accomplish everything we should. Many of us feel stretched to the limit by our responsibilities and obligations at work and at home. Because there's always too much to do, we feel stressed, anxious, tired, or just worn out. In the process, our neurotransmitters and neuronutrients take a beating.

To restore balance and improve our moods and behavior, it's crucial that we reduce the stress in our lives and make more time for ourselves. What exactly is balance? I think of it as maintaining a degree of equilibrium between the things you do for other people (such as your boss, spouse, and children) and things you need to do to be a physically and mentally healthy person.

I have found that three basic lifestyle strategies will help you to create a buffer zone against stress and will give you time to recharge yourself.

These three strategies are:

1. Defining your personal boundaries

2. Reshuffling your priorities

3. Uncluttering and simplifying your life

The strategies are relatively simple, and for some people they will seem obvious. Unfortunately, we don't always see the obvious—or act on it—especially when we feel stressed. Combined with my supplement and dietary recommendations, these strategies will allow you to create more time for satisfying activities, reduce the amount of stress in your life, and improve your moods and behavior.

I urge you not to use this newfound time to get more work done at the office or tackle a few more chores at home. That would be self-defeating. While neuronutrient supplements can boost your resistance to stress and improve your moods and behavior, they do have their limitations. It is more holistic and effective when you simultaneously modify the lifestyle patterns that contribute to stress.

Your Personal Boundaries

The pressures of modern life tempt people to regularly violate the personal boundaries of other people. We feel stressed when someone intrudes on our personal space. We need to define and maintain our personal boundaries to prevent this from happening. We can do this firmly but politely.

What exactly are these boundaries? Personal boundaries are both the physical and the emotional spaces around us. They are also the limits we set to prevent other people from annoying us or from trampling on our privacy, time, or emotional sensitivities. When we don't set these boundaries, we allow ourselves to be taken advantage of and to become stressed. Following are examples of how personal space is violated, with suggestions on how you can define and maintain your boundaries.

How Boundaries Are Commonly Violated

Animal studies have long shown that overcrowding breeds aggressive behavior. In such situations, the animals cannot maintain their normal territories—that is, boundaries. You know what it feels like when someone stands too close to you in line at the bank or the supermarket. That other person has entered your personal space, and you're no longer comfortable. The person seems to be "breathing down your neck." This expression refers to a predator that is too close. Another example is a man who pressures his wife to have intercourse when she's not in the mood. He is violating her physical and emotional boundaries by literally trying to enter her space when she doesn't want him to.

A friend, Malcolm, once told me about a girlfriend who kept violating his boundaries. He needed a little space for himself and asked her to leave him alone in his home office for a while. She followed the letter of his request but not the spirit of it: she stood by the doorway and kept trying to have a conversation with him. She was violating Malcolm's boundaries.

As a group, advertisers are among the most aggressive and relentless of personal boundary violators. In the United States, people are subjected to an estimated three thousand advertising messages each day.

Quick Tip

Visualize . . . Something Better

If you can daydream, you can enjoy the benefits of the stress-reducing activity called guided imagery.

What's the difference? Daydreaming often amounts to a fantasy, which can be either relaxing or distracting. Guided imagery follows several methodical steps to reduce anxiety and stress.

Like meditation, guided imagery leads to a more relaxed feeling. Guided imagery uses specific mental images, called visualizations. You can follow these steps, but here are a couple of tips. One, the more realistic your mental image, the better your response will be. Two, find a quiet place to visualize.

First, picture a place you really like. For example, it might be a forest or a beach.

Second, be sure to take slow, deep breaths.

Third, imagine what the place sounds like. Try to hear the sound of a breeze through the trees or of waves washing up on the beach. Use all five of your senses—hearing, sight, touch, taste, and smell—to visualize.

Fourth, visualize the effect on your body.

Allow ten to fifteen minutes for each visualization. You'll get better with practice.

Many people use guided visualization to stimulate their immune systems or as a healing method to overcome diseases. Serious diseases can contribute to anxiety or depression. If you have a chronic disease, such as cancer, you might visualize immune cells eating away at your tumor.

Boundary violations are why so many people hate telemarketers—their telephone calls violate our space during dinner or while we're watching television at home.

Our boundaries are violated in still other ways. For example, parents might allow their children and their toys full reign of the house, instead of maintaining a well-defined "adults only" space. Similarly, some couples may not recognize that each person has his or her own individual activities to pursue, such as hobbies or meeting with friends. Couples cannot do everything together; they must allow time for each person to be an individual.

How to Define Your Personal Boundaries

Many people don't understand the importance of personal boundaries, even though they may feel vague discomfort when their boundaries are violated. Sometimes people allow it to happen because they have regularly been victimized, because they are afraid of hurting another person's feelings, or because they are simply too overwhelmed to stop and think about the many violations they endure.

It's important to set our boundaries and not let other people cross them. Boundary violations are one sign of an unhealthy relationship. Consider the case of Jeff. He was dating a high-maintenance woman who required an extraordinary amount of personal attention. Nancy abhorred silence and always wanted Jeff to engage in conversation. He could not read through a page in a book without Nancy interrupting him. Even when Jeff was at work, Nancy called several times a day. He became increasingly resentful until he heard, for the first time, about the idea of personal boundaries. He immediately realized that he needed to reestablish his boundaries for work and down time. When Jeff politely but firmly set his boundaries, Nancy argued with him and tried to make him feel guilty. Although Jeff loved Nancy, he eventually had to end the relationship to maintain his boundaries and preserve the essence of who he was.

Learn to say no. People who have difficulty saying no are often the ones who invite boundary violations. They may say yes because they want to please or not offend another person. By saying yes, however, they end up sacrificing their own time and energy for other people. Saying no (kindly but firmly) is often a way of defining a boundary. Other words that work just as well include "No thanks," "I can't," "Can't do that," or an incredulous "Excuse me?" Offering too many explanations may be a sign that you feel defensive and guilty.

Draw the line at work. Bosses and coworkers frequently violate our boundaries. Occasional overtime may be a necessity in today's work environment, but working long hours, even with great compensation, robs you of time to rest, recharge yourself, and maintain balance in your life. No one would argue that workaholics lead balanced lives.

The trick is to tactfully establish your boundaries without getting fired.

First, the sooner you set your boundaries, the better off you'll be in the long run. That's because you have set a precedent and aren't trying to change one.

Second, if your boundaries have to be soft because of a particular work environment, try negotiating to get something in return. For example, if you're told during a job interview that periodic overtime is a requirement, ask whether you can trade it for comp time (time off).

Third, not every boundary issue is with a boss or a supervisor. Sexual harassment is a boundary violation. Office complainers violate the boundaries of coworkers who want to get their work done. Define your boundary to avoid distractions, and do your job.

Detach and distance yourself. In the original *Star Trek* television series, Mr. Spock used his emotional detachment to stay calm in the most stressful situations. His detachment often exasperated his more emotional colleagues, but Mr. Spock frequently found the solution to problems by separating his thinking from his emotions.

Detachment is a powerful way to protect your boundaries and avoid a lot of emotional anguish. The essence of detachment is not to react emotionally. You don't have to be as aloof as Mr. Spock, and you can express some empathy. By restraining your emotions, however, you're less likely to arouse emotional reactions on the part of other people.

One detachment technique requires reframing how you see another person's words and actions: don't take his or her words personally.

Instead, accept that the words reflect that person's inner turmoil or frustration with life.

It takes a little effort to be good at this type of reframing and detachment, but you can practice it while commuting. When another driver honks at you or speeds past you impatiently, remind yourself that you haven't done anything wrong (that is, unless you've clearly done something wrong!). You were driving conscientiously and at the speed limit. Recognize that the other driver's horn honking and speeding reflect his or her impatience and stress, not something you did.

Allow yourself down time. Everyone needs down time to reflect, process experiences, and think about the past and the future. Without down time, life becomes little more than running on a big hamster wheel—you're on the move, but you aren't doing anything meaningful.

Down time is usually (though not always) solitary time. It can involve reading, gardening, writing, painting, meditating, praying, thinking about your life, or performing any other activity that helps to recenter you with what you consider important. You can have this type of solitary down time even if your significant other is in the same room; the key is that he or she not interrupt your down time.

Quick Tip

To Relax, Do Something Routine

So many of us have jobs in which we must be unfailingly productive or creative. We might like the challenges and the pay of our jobs, but these demands often stress us.

Doing something routine, even for a half hour, can be a powerful stress reliever. Repetitive tasks can often induce a meditative state. One task is filing. Another is organizing. Yet another is cleaning your desk. If you're at home, slice, chop, or dice some food. Rather than wasting your time, these activities can actually help to clear your mind.

Honor the Sabbath or create one for yourself. In ancient times, the Sabbath was intended as a day of rest after working hard for six days. These days, it's difficult to give yourself a full day for the Sabbath—after all, when you're not working, you're likely catching up with household-related chores. Yet adopting the idea of a Sabbath is a worthy counterbalance to the amount of time that work demands of us.

If you are a religious person, honor at least part of your Sabbath, and do a little more than merely go to your house of worship and pray. Take some time to read and reflect on your life, family, and friends. Consider ways to express your gratitude for what's right in your life—expressions of gratitude are a great stress reliever. If you are not religious, create your own Sabbath as a contemplative day or half-day of calming music, creative activities, or relaxing time with a loved one. These activities will recenter you and restore your energy levels before you return to work.

Reshuffle Your Priorities

Depending on your family and neighbors, living in overcrowded conditions may or may not contribute to your feeling edgy and aggressive. Living an overcrowded life, however, will definitely leave you feeling stressed and overwhelmed. When your plate is full with work and home activities, you're desperately trying to complete tasks rather than deciding whether you should even be doing them.

Consider, once again, the negative aspects of multitasking. Multitasking is a sign that you have no clear priorities and you're trying to do everything at once. By its very nature, multitasking prevents people

Quick Tip

Sounds That Soothe Your Mind and Mood

Sounds affect all of us. Just think about how you feel when a car horn rattles you or the way a Vivaldi concerto relaxes you.

For forty years, the Monroe Institute in Faber, Virginia, has researched how specific sonic frequencies affect thinking and emotions. The institute sells CDs designed to enhance relaxation, mental sharpness, and restful sleep.

According to Brian Dailey, M.D., of the Rochester School of Medicine and Dentistry in upstate New York, certain tonal patterns promote relaxation and sleep, whereas others encourage mental clarity and concentration. Dailey asks all of his surgical patients to listen to specific CDs that are designed to reduce pain. He has found that patients who listen to the CDs need less pain medication and recover more quickly after surgery.

According to an article in the journal *Alternative and Complementary Therapies*, these CDs are best listened to with stereo headphones that send one tonal pattern through one ear and another through the other ear. Together, they set up a third tone within the brain, leading to "hemispheric synchronization," or simply Hemi-Sync. For more information, visit www.monroeinstitute.org.

from giving their full attention to any single task. The solution is to reshuffle your priorities and decide what to do first, second, and third.

Granted, it's not always easy to realign your priorities at work and home, especially if your boss wants to juggle multiple tasks simultaneously. To shuffle your priorities, you must take a moment to consider what you're doing and must be willing to make some changes. And for many people, changing their routines is uncomfortable, if not a little scary.

Make "To Do" Lists. Lists are wonderful organizational tools—they can help you decide what's important and what isn't, as well as help you remember what you must do. Make two lists for what you have to do today or tomorrow, one for work and another for home-related activities (such as grocery shopping).

Writing your to do list should take no more than a few minutes. Prioritize each item on your list by numbering it, then transcribe the prioritized list in numerical order to another slip of paper. Do the same for your home-related chores.

There's a chance that you won't finish everything on your lists for today, so transfer your uncompleted tasks to tomorrow's list. Do the same each day. If the same task keeps getting moved each day for a week, consider whether you actually need to do it or whether it belongs on a broader to do list without any particular deadline. In making lists, always bear two things in mind. One, what *must* you do today? Two, what do you *not* have to do today?

Unclutter and Simplify Your Life

It's often hard to make time in our lives or figure out what's important when we're surrounded by too much clutter. Clutter is a distraction that keeps us from clearly focusing on more meaningful and less stressful activities. We must get rid of what isn't really necessary.

Our lives are cluttered with all sorts of things—clothing, electronic gadgets, tools, videos, and antique collections, to name just a few. The simplicity movement and simplicity circles have grown as a response to a society that seems to be on a continual spending spree. Rather than being part of a back-to-the-woods movement, the desire for simplicity stems from a number of basic ideas. One is that less actually translates into more. If we devote more time to meaningful activities, we'll be less susceptible to the lure of owning the latest expensive gadget, which will be obsolete in a year. We'll also do a better job of saving money.

Like overeaters who eat out of boredom, overshoppers often shop to fill a void in their lives. The act of shopping—driving to and then perusing products at the mall—feels like a productive activity. Yet shopping is more like having a chocolate bar—it feels good for a few moments but doesn't usually do much to enhance your life.

Distinguish between needs and wants. Do you understand the difference between your needs and your wants? The basic necessities of life are food, shelter, and income. Wants are everything else—discretionary purchases or activities. That doesn't mean all wants are bad. After all, there's no point in being a miser and dying with a million dollars under your mattress. It's all about striking a balance. Along the way, though, it helps to recognize whether you are buying something to fulfill a need or a want.

People who spend too much money on their wants may sacrifice their long-term ability to pay for their needs. Reports have consistently found that relatively few Americans bother saving any substantial amount of money. Instead, they succumb to buying the latest consumer products and often carry considerable high-interest credit card debt.

Control your shopping. How can you change shopaholic behavior? According to Mike Millard, a friend and one of the simplicity gurus in Tucson, Arizona, it helps to follow five steps.

- When you do have to go shopping, always use a shopping list.
- If you're tempted to make an impulse purchase, ask yourself whether you can live without the product.
- Resist the seduction of advertising. The whole point of advertising is to make you believe that you must buy a particular product, whether you need it or not.
- Don't buy something because you're afraid to say no. The salesperson is not your friend; his or her job is to sell you something.

- Finally, appreciate what you already have.

Declutter the rest of your life. Simplifying your life doesn't apply only to consumer goods. If your social schedule often leaves you feeling burned out, you may have to declutter your social life. Ask yourself whether all your activities and friends enhance your quality of life or leave you feeling stretched thin and tired. If those activities are taking a toll on you, it's time to reshuffle your priorities.

Create a More Balanced Life

After you start to firm up your boundaries, set priorities, and reduce clutter in your life, you will have more time and space to further modify and improve the quality of your life and your resistance to stress. The principal ideas here are

- Get enough rest
- Build your resilience
- Learn to appreciate being in the moment
- Learn to laugh about the everyday silliness in life
- Deal with your negative emotions
- Cultivate healthy relationships

This is also where I part company with many of my colleagues who think that taking supplements (or medications) is all you need to do to improve your moods and behavior. As beneficial as good nutrition and supplements are, they cannot by themselves correct dysfunctional or problematic relationships with other people. Bad moods and behavior are almost always distorted responses to stressful situations. Changing your environment or your responses to the environment reduces your stress load, and that lessens the impact on your neurotransmitters and frees up neuronutrients to support good moods.

Get Enough Rest

So many things interfere with our ability to get a good night's sleep. Sometimes anxiety keeps us awake at night. Other times, our dietary habits, such as drinking too many caffeine-containing beverages, make us too keyed up to sleep. Heartburn is often caused by consuming soft drinks or processed foods, especially in the evening, and can disrupt sleep. Sleep apnea, which is common among overweight, diabetic, and prediabetic people, interferes with normal breathing and interrupts sleep. The consequence is that we go to bed tired, wake up tired, and muddle through the day feeling tired, cranky, and like zombies.

J. Todd Arnedt, Ph.D., of the University of Michigan, has found that working very long hours produces the same slow reflexes and poor judgment as when we drink too much alcohol. A lack of restful sleep increases levels of cortisol, the body's chief stress hormone, which helps to store fat around the belly. As you already know, being overweight is a sign of prediabetes and possibly full-blown diabetes, and the associated fluctuations in blood sugar can affect both moods and thinking processes.

To improve your restful sleep, consider adopting some of the following habits.

Reduce your consumption of caffeinated drinks. These beverages include coffee, black tea, and cola and many noncola (e.g., Mountain Dew) soft drinks. If you need a little caffeine to perk you up, try one or two cups of green tea. The L-theanine in green tea improves mental focus while also moderating the stimulating effect of caffeine. Avoid drinking any caffeinated beverages later than two hours after you wake up.

Cut back on sugars and refined carbs. These foods include sweets, candies, energy bars, cereals, pastas, breads, and pizza. Sugars and refined carbs are used to make many processed foods, so you will have to give up most foods in boxes, jars, and other packages. These foods trigger rapid increases and decreases in blood sugar, which leave you feeling tired and wanting caffeine as a stimulant.

Don't eat late dinners, and don't eat any food after 7:30 p.m. Eating a late dinner can result in either low or high blood sugar levels by morning, which will diminish your energy levels and make you dependent on the transient stimulating effects of caffeine and sugar. If you work the swing or the graveyard shift, avoid eating anything for two to three hours before going to sleep, although drinking water is perfectly fine.

Go to bed at a consistent time. We often push ourselves on workdays, staying up too late and waking up early. Come the weekend, we sleep late at least one day. In the process, we go from feeling sleep deprived to sleep saturated. It's far better to wake up and go to sleep at consistent times. Don't vary your wake and sleep times by more than one hour on your days off.

Prepare for sleep. Brush your teeth and wash your face early in the evening. (Doing so will also discourage you from eating later that evening.) About one hour before you go to sleep, turn the lights low, turn off the television, and read. You can also listen to soft, relaxing music during this time. If there's a late-evening television show that you'd like to see, tape it and watch it another night.

Keep the television out of your bedroom. Some people enjoy watching television or reading a book, a magazine, or a newspaper in bed before turning off the lights. The bedroom should really be for just three activities: sex, pillow talk, and sleep. Read or watch television in another room.

Keep your laptop computer out of the bedroom. It's becoming more common for couples to work on their laptop computers in the bedroom before dozing off. Although some people think working side by side in bed is a form of intimacy, it's really a sign of stress, obsessive-compulsive behavior, and a lack of boundaries between personal and professional lives. If you must work, go into your home office. But it would probably be much better for you to shut off the computer and to touch and talk with your significant other—and maybe even be a little romantic.

Arrange and decorate your bedroom for relaxation. Some people have messy bedrooms with poorly arranged furniture. While you don't have to adopt the Chinese principles of feng shui, your bedroom should be neat, and you shouldn't have to dodge furniture or other objects to reach your bed. Bedroom clutter often reflects a cluttered life and mind, and

Quick Tip

Insulate Yourself from Noise

Noise is a stress. Depending on where you live, you may often be exposed to the sound of traffic, airplanes, construction, and lawn mowers. Noise is distracting, it gets on your nerves, and it can make you irritable. Being regularly exposed to noise can also triple your risk of having a heart attack. That was the finding of a European study in which researchers compared men and women living in noisy and quiet settings.

It's important to distance or insulate yourself from noise. Doing so helps you to maintain some of your personal boundaries, which noise violates. Going for a walk or a hike in nature is one way to escape noise. If you have a private office, close the door to insulate yourself. At home, you can turn off the television. When you're driving, listen to soft music or simply be alone with your thoughts.

that means you may have too much going on inside your head to settle down for a restful sleep. Also, consider painting at least one wall a light green, lavender, or mauve; these colors can help to soothe your nerves.

Build Your Resilience

We don't hear the word *resilience* very often, but it's an important stress-resisting personality trait. Resilience is the ability of an object to return to its original shape after being bent or stretched—or stressed in some other way. A rubber ball may not be as strong as a steel ball, but the rubber ball is far more resilient.

Dealing effectively with change, disappointment, and adversity is central to being resilient. So is learning from negative experiences and following the adage of "turning lemons into lemonade." Change is scary for many people—it's full of unknowns—but learning how to adapt to change (instead of fighting it) increases resilience.

There are several ways to foster greater resilience, although these changes take time. Don't be afraid to take baby steps at first.

Step out of your comfort zone. Given our druthers, most of us prefer to follow our personal routines. After all, predictability provides a sense of familiarity and security. Yet you can learn to step out of your comfort zone in small and safe ways. When you find that little changes don't

hurt—and might actually be rewarding—you build your self-confidence.
That's good because self-confidence
and resilience go hand in hand. As you
become more self-confident in dealing
with change, your resilience increases.
So stretch yourself a little and do things
you haven't done before. For example,
consider going to a modern dance performance, an art museum, a rodeo, or a
country music concert.

*Pay attention and learn from your
experiences.* You've probably heard the
phrase "Those who cannot learn from
history are doomed to repeat it,"
penned by George Santayana, a His-
panic American philosopher. Although
people often quote Santayana in terms
of politicians making the same mistakes over and over again, the same
idea applies to your individual life. Paying attention to and learning
from your experiences—what you have done right and what you have
done wrong—gives you a broader perspective to interpret what goes
on around you. These qualities are particularly important if you tend to
repeat the same negative patterns in your life, such as in relationships
at home or at work.

> ### Quick Tip
>
> **Better Breathing Leads
> to a Better Mood**
> When we're stressed, we tend
> to hold our breath or take very
> small breaths of air. Taking
> three or four slow, very deep
> breaths can help you to loosen
> up and disengage from a
> stressful situation. You can
> adopt and simplify some of the
> techniques of meditation. Sit
> upright in a chair with your feet
> flat on the floor. This breathing
> exercise uses the word *healing*.
> Inhale slowly and deeply while
> you stretch out the syllable
> "hee." Next, exhale slowly while
> saying "aahhh." As you finish
> exhaling, think "ling" to yourself
> or say it aloud. Do this breath-
> ing exercise several times a day.
> You'll become quieter and
> more relaxed as you repeat it.

Appreciate Being in the Moment

You may have heard the phrases "Be mindful" or "Be in the moment"
and wondered what they meant. These sayings mean being aware of the
immediacy of people, surroundings, and events. In other words, you
focus on the present without being distracted, don't dwell on the past,
and don't fantasize or have expectations about the future.

I'll give you an example of how people are *not* mindful. At least
once a week, while walking across a parking lot or through a store, I

inadvertently startle people who are busy talking on their cell phones. They're so absorbed in their phone conversations that they are not aware of other people or vehicles and are extremely vulnerable to being mugged or hit by cars. They are not being mindful or in the moment.

Train yourself to focus. With all the distractions in our lives, as well as with the pressure to multitask, it's often difficult to stay in the present. It requires being fully conscious of your surroundings and focusing on what you're doing, not on the end result. Focusing is a lot like paying attention, except that your field of vision is much narrower, on one person or one task.

To be mindful, let's say, of another person or a conversation, resist the temptation to say what's on your mind. Instead, pay attention to what the other person is saying, and rephrase his or her words to ensure that you understand them. Instead of interrupting or interjecting, wait for a natural pause and segue in the conversation. To be mindful when you're driving, focus on your car, traffic patterns, and road conditions. If you're using your cell phone or opening mail while driving, you are not being mindful—you are distracted, and that increases your risk of injuring yourself or other people in an accident.

As another example, many men see sexual intercourse as the payoff for being romantic. This view focuses on one end result and prevents men from being in the moment. If you are in the moment, you can enjoy a lot of small payoffs. First, be mindful of your girlfriend's or wife's feelings. If you're in the moment, you will pay attention and follow her cues as to how intimate she wants to become. Many if not most women take longer than men to warm up physically. Being in the moment allows you to relish kissing and touching for hours because you've detached yourself from where these activities might lead. For many women (though not all) this slow-and-easy, in-the-moment approach is one of the biggest turn-ons. (Guys, take note!) Kissing and cuddling are a lot of fun, and if you think about it, they extend and heighten the pleasure of lovemaking beyond that of a brief orgasm.

Dispense with your expectations. We often have certain expectations in life—that we'll go on a thrilling date, get a spectacular Christmas gift, or win the lottery. The trouble is that people or experiences often fail to meet our expectations. When that happens, we may feel disappointed or depressed. If we can suspend our expectations, even for a little while, we're more likely to feel better about the outcome. Expectations are often nothing more than wishful thinking, and they distract us from being in the moment.

Find ways to recenter yourself. Many people turn to meditation and yoga as a way to relax and remove stress from their bodies. For some people,

Quick Tip

Keep a Journal

Journaling has become an increasingly popular way of furthering emotional and physical healing. We all have a need to express ourselves. When we can't safely say what we're feeling or what's on our mind, or when no one is interested in listening, we feel isolated and vulnerable. The situation even affects our physical health. All of our unexpressed feelings and thoughts eat away at us like an emotional cancer.

In one study, published in the *Journal of the American Medical Association*, researchers asked patients with asthma or rheumatoid arthritis to write about either their most stressful life experiences or emotionally neutral things they've experienced over the course of several months. People who wrote about stressful experiences had almost a one-fifth reduction in symptoms. Those who wrote about nonstressful experiences had no improvement. Writing about stressful experiences was a way of getting them out of their system.

You don't have to be a writer to benefit from keeping a journal. It's a little like writing a letter, and you can either keep what you've written or eventually throw it out. If you've never written much beyond a grocery list, here are some tips.

One, you can write with a pen and paper or on a computer. Choose whichever is easiest for you.

Two, don't worry about grammar, spelling, or organization. No one will grade you. It's all right to use incomplete sentences.

Three, write about something that bothers you. Again, it's okay to describe feelings or thoughts you have because no one else will ever read what you've written. (If there's any chance that another person might snoop and find your journal, put it in a safe place.)

Four, add the date to what you've written. You might want to review your journal entries over a number of months.

Five, if you've reviewed your writing over several months and found that the tone is negative, give yourself a new writing assignment: figure out how you can make things in your life better.

however, the Eastern approaches to meditation and yoga are a bit too exotic and alien. If you're not comfortable with a particular practice, it will add stress rather than remove it. Quiet prayers can be meditative, as can reading the Bible or self-help psychology books. I have one friend who finds that long horseback rides in the desert induce a thoughtful meditative state. Creative pursuits, such as writing or painting or hobbies, can also help you to recenter yourself.

You can adopt any number of nontraditional meditative activities. It took me many years to realize that photographing old buildings and desert scenes was my own meditative experience. I photograph slowly (with a large manual camera) and literally focus my attention on an object—the essence of meditation. Sweeping the floor, slowly carving a piece of wood, slicing or dicing food by hand, or even cleaning the house can be a meditative experience. The key is to allow yourself to be so absorbed in the activity that you forget about time.

Accept and Laugh about the Everyday Silliness in Life

Laughter can have a powerful and positive effect on both your physical and your mental health. Years ago, when the writer Norman Cousins was bedridden with a serious illness, he used vitamin C and laughter—watching old Three Stooges movies—to recover. Laughing is good for the heart, improves overall circulation, and reduces blood sugar levels. It also eases muscle tension and encourages deep, healthy breathing.

Having a good laugh—what one researcher calls "mirthful," or playful, laughter—can produce significant changes in neurohormones and neurotransmitters. Lee S. Berk, M.D., of the Loma Linda University School of Medicine, California, found that laughing led to significant reductions in hormones and stress-related neurotransmitters. In later experiments, Berk reported that laughter boosted the activity of immune cells, which help you fight colds, flus, and other diseases.

Laughter is a good way to gauge the mental health of other people, and I often say that you can't trust anyone who doesn't laugh. It's also important to pay attention to what someone finds funny. Racist and sexist humor is offensive and says a lot about the person making the wisecracks—and about the people laughing at those jokes. Conversely, wit or puns reflect a sharp perceptiveness about the common absurdities of life.

Quick Tip

Touching Other People's Lives

Alternative and complementary practitioners know the benefits of therapeutic massage, but a little-known nonmassage touching technique can also do wonders for both body and mind. It's called Bio-Touch and it's easy to learn.

Bio-Touch uses a very light two-finger touch, called a butterfly touch because it's that light. At the Bio-Touch Center in Tucson, Arizona, teacher and practitioner Paul Bucky makes no therapeutic claims for the technique but says that people report feeling less anxious and depressed and more energetic.

How could such a light touch produce such benefits? Studies by Kenna Stephenson, M.D., of the University of Texas, Tyler, have found that the Bio-Touch technique activates several genes involved in immunity and longevity, while also shutting off genes involved in dementia and cancer.

The Bio-Touch organization is nonprofit, and payment for touch sessions in Tucson is on a donation-only basis. You can learn the technique from information at www.justtouch.com or by calling the Bio-Touch center at 520-751-7751.

Bucky does believe that a lot of social and psychological problems are related to people not touching one another. These days, even doctors are reluctant to touch patients, and many people in general hesitate to touch others because of the fear that their actions may be misinterpreted.

One of the funniest people I've ever met is Carl A. Hammerslag, M.D., a psychiatrist and author who lives and works in Phoenix, Arizona. In a presentation at the University of Arizona, he described how he and Hunter "Patch" Adams, M.D., once donned costumes and took a trip to a shopping mall. Hammerslag dressed up as a toilet bowl and a seat, which he said was appropriate as a psychiatrist—"because patients are always dumping on me!" Children at the mall thought the sight of a person dressed up as a toilet was absolutely hilarious.

Deal with Your Negative Emotions

If you consider the sources of the conflicts and the irritations in your life, you'll realize that nearly all stem from your relationships with other people. These relationships might be with your spouse, your coworkers, your buddies, your children, your parents, your supervisors, or strangers you encounter in stores or on the road.

The negative emotions that you repeatedly brood over or act out are what many people call "emotional baggage." This baggage is likely related to past hurts—perhaps the unfairness of a parent, a put-down by a romantic interest, or a disparaging comment from a boss. These events might also persist in your mind because of the I-should-have-done syndrome, in which you later realize that you might have been more assertive in speaking out or acting on your own behalf.

Negative emotions can churn inside a person and affect moods for months or years, and they can resurface and destroy relationships. If you resent something another person did to you, you pay a psychological price with negative emotions weighing on you—and draining your neuronutrients. Your resentment bothers no one else. It is far better to let go of the negative emotions. To do this, you sometimes have to remind yourself that, as an example, a crude comment from a coworker almost always says more about that person than it does about you.

Anger is another common negative emotion. Psychologists know that anger is not a primary emotion. Rather, it is a secondary emotion that develops in response to a primary emotion, such as feeling hurt or frustrated. If you often feel angry, give some thought to what triggered your anger. To gain an understanding of their emotions, people can sometimes process their feelings by talking with friends, reading self-help psychology books, or talking with a counselor or a psychologist. This type of emotional processing reduces their emotional turbulence and stress.

Quick Tip

Learn to Say "I" Instead of "You"

As anyone who has been in an argument knows, it's easy to make accusations and to attack the other person. It even feels good to let all of your built-up resentment explode. Unfortunately, "You did this" and "You did that" are worn-out refrains, and blaming the other person rarely resolves anything.

Instead, therapists recommend using the pronoun "I" instead of "you." It takes a little practice, but it fundamentally alters how people express their grievances to each other.

The idea behind "I" is relatively simple. When you say "You did ...," you're making an accusation, and it's natural for the other person to feel defensive, as well as compelled to toss his or her own salvo at you. When, however, you say, "I feel ..." (such as "I feel hurt when you ignore me"), you're expressing your own feeling. Without accusations or attacks, it's less tempting for the other person to counterattack.

How you can let go of negative emotions. To let go of your negative emotions, you first have to take responsibility, or ownership, for your words and actions. This means not blaming other people for your frustrations, but instead recognizing the mistakes you've made or the situations you've gotten yourself into. Taking ownership can be difficult because many of us have grown up believing we'll be punished for what we've done wrong, and we often lie or deny to avoid punishment. When you're wrong, admit that you're wrong and say you're sorry.

With life's trials and tribulations, it's often easy to get stuck in a negative frame of mind. One way to counterbalance this negativity is to allow one minute each day for thinking about what's right in your life. As children, many of us did this with a bedtime prayer to thank the Lord for everything that was good in our lives. It could simply be a minute-long expression of gratitude. (See the upcoming section on gratitude.)

Improve your self-talk. Some people say negative things about themselves in their minds. Examples of negative self-talk include such thoughts as "I can't ever do things right," "I'm not doing it fast enough," and "What's wrong with me?" Work on changing these negative feelings into positive affirmations, such as "I'll do it right, even if it takes me a little longer at first."

Stop trying to control other people. If you look for the source of most relationship conflicts, and the resulting resentment and anger, you'll usually come to two underlying problems: one is the desire to control what another person thinks or does, and the other is poor communication. Often, the two are intertwined.

Sometimes the desire to control is so ingrained that people have difficulty understanding it. An anal person is a controller, and he or she usually controls by micromanaging other people. People may try to control others through various forms of bullying, such as suggesting that others are stupid if they have opposing political views. Behavior that is mentally or physically abusive reflects a dangerous type of controller.

Sometimes, people control others indirectly, such as through passive-aggressive resistance or manipulation. People who are passive-aggressive rarely describe their true feelings or wants. Instead, they might use flattery or feign some type of weakness to get other people to do what they want.

The desire to control others stems from our individual egos and our self-centeredness—and the unreasonable belief that people should do what we want. If you are a controller, you want people to behave or do things in certain ways—namely, the ways you would like them done. This tendency includes some degree of obsessive-compulsive behavior.

Consider Trish's story. After many failed relationships, she couldn't give up her control issues. As she once told me (a casual friend), "There's no problem finding a guy who likes to do the things I like doing. The problem I have is in the details, such as the fact that he stacks the dishwasher differently from the way I do it."

In such situations, psychologists and counselors commonly tell their clients this: you can't control another person, and the only person you can control is you. To change another person or situation, you have to first change yourself. For Trish, the best solution (silly as it might sound) might have been for her to express her frustration and to come to some agreement on how to stack the dishwasher.

Like it or not, you simply have to accept the fact that most people will do things differently from the way you do. It takes genuine practice— and often a very deep breath—to make a conscious decision not to react. Gently joking about the other person's foibles often helps, as long as you can tolerate kidding in return. There are few things that work better than simple acceptance, though.

Express gratitude and forgiveness. Gratitude and forgiveness are two antidotes for resentments and grudges. Think of gratitude as taking a moment to appreciate people who have meant a lot to you or have done a lot for you at some time in your life. Similarly, think of forgiveness as a form of personal absolution for people who have intentionally or inadvertently hurt you. The positive nature of these emotions will help you to vanquish self-harmful negative emotions and buoy your mood-enhancing neurotransmitters.

As you've already learned, moods have a powerful effect on your overall biochemistry. Negative moods increase the secretion of your stress hormones, which reduces your resistance to disease and slows healing.

In contrast, gratitude and forgiveness are positive acts that create an almost meditative mood. At the Bright Spot for Health, a nutritionally oriented medical clinic in Wichita, Kansas, patients, staff, and visitors can walk along a "gratitude trail" that wraps around a tranquil pond. Along the trail, people have placed marble plaques or red bricks with brief statements of gratitude for people who have meant a lot to them. There are also stone benches to sit on and to contemplate people in your life.

We all make mistakes in life. Although I am not a Catholic, I do marvel at the concept of confession, after which a person is forgiven for his or her sins. That type of forgiveness can relieve people of a burdensome guilt. When you as an individual forgive someone, you let go of your resentment and other negative emotions that are tied to what that person did to hurt you. When you forgive yourself, you shed guilt and anger.

How Jonathan Recovered from a Difficult Relationship

Jonathan had gone through a bitter divorce and then found himself in an emotionally up-and-down relationship for three years. Although both he and his girlfriend wanted the relationship to work, the regular disagreements, arguments, and stresses wore him down.

Toward the end of the relationship, Jonathan's right arm became extremely sore. A counselor pointed out that the right arm is a person's "giving arm," and Jonathan gave too much of himself to the relationship.

A nutritionally oriented physician saw how the stresses in Jonathan's life probably depleted his vitamin B6 levels. Symptomatically, the sore arm had similarities to carpal tunnel syndrome, which can be helped with vitamin B6. The physician also knew that vitamin B6 was needed to make neurotransmitters, such as serotonin, that help people resist and recover from stress.

When Jonathan began taking high doses of vitamin B6 (along with a high-potency B-complex supplement), his arm started to feel better. After several months, it was almost back to normal.

Cultivate Healthy Relationships

With half of all marriages in the United States (including my own) ending in divorce, it's painfully obvious that people have difficulty cultivating and maintaining healthy relationships. Nor is it any easier to foster a healthy relationship with a boss, a subordinate, or one's children. A good relationship requires dealing with negative feelings we've accumulated over the years and having honest, tactful communication with another person. Yet differences of opinion are inevitable, and most of us know that it's much easier to avoid uncomfortable subjects—until our resentments explode in anger. Of course, resentment and anger take their toll on our neurotransmitters and neuronutrients.

It takes time, hard work, and a conscientious approach to resolve the inevitable disagreements in a fair and equitable way and to know when to ignore some issues (such as the other person's quirks). Healthy relationships can occasionally be scary because they require that we reveal our weaknesses, which makes us emotionally vulnerable. We've learned that some people will exploit or abuse our weaknesses, thus we're cautious about what we reveal to other people. Although I will focus on romantic relationships in this section, you can apply most of the principles to other types of interactions.

Follow these agreements for healthy conversations. The Conversation Café concept, which began in Seattle and is now active in many cities, revolves around small groups of people engaged in thoughtful discussions, not debates. Each conversation focuses on a particular topic and lasts for about one and one-half hours. Before the actual conversation begins, participants agree to honor and follow several ground rules. These ground rules are good to follow in life.

The exact wording of the Conversation Café agreements varies somewhat between locations. The following agreements are not copyrighted, and I've borrowed them from the Tucson Conversation Cafés. I try to follow these agreements when talking with and listening to other people.

- Listen with respect.
- Seek to understand rather than to persuade.
- Suspend judgment as best you can.

- Invite and honor diversity of opinion.

- Speak from the heart with personal meaning.

- Go for honesty and depth without going on and on.

If there is a Conversation Café in your city, I encourage you to attend some of its discussions. You can find out more about the organization and its locations at www.conversationcafe.org. I found that the Conversation Café experience reminded me of and reinforced sound principles for great conversations. You can easily apply all of these agreements to your conversations with other people. Of these, listening is of paramount importance.

Learn to listen and validate. John Gray, Ph.D., the author of the Mars-Venus relationship books, has often pointed out the differences between how men and women communicate. Men usually have a clear linear purpose in communicating, whereas women tend to be more nonlinear in conversation. Men frequently assume that when a woman describes a problem, she is actually asking for a solution, but sometimes women just want to air their thoughts and feelings. When a woman talks with a man, he often becomes restless with the lack of a clear direction, looks at his watch, interrupts by suggesting a solution, or ends up dominating the conversation.

Half of any good conversation is listening—just shutting up for a while. Really listening and occasionally acknowledging or restating what the other person says amount to a validation of that person's experiences, whether it was a bad day at work or some other issue. When you're upset or feel that you have to vent your feelings, you want someone else to listen and acknowledge your experience, not give you a solution. (Suggesting a solution might be appropriate and well received later.)

Acknowledging another person's experience is the essence of validation. You may not totally agree with that person's views, but you haven't experienced what that person has, either. Allowing people to safely express their feelings without fear of criticism or attack is one reason why the Conversation Café concept has been so successful. In today's acrimonious and divisive world of red and blue states, of one social or political group pitted against another, it's a wonderful experience to connect with the similarities we all share.

Listen without being reactive. In his book *The Lost Art of Listening*, psychologist Michael P. Nichols, Ph.D., explores how people have lost the ability to listen to each other. There are many reasons for this loss. When a person is criticized, it's natural to go on the offensive, and most spouses know the emotional weaknesses of their significant other.

Part of the reason is also social. We are often so time-stressed that we feel as if we don't have time to genuinely listen to another person. And part of the reason is nutritional. When we're stressed and not eating healthful foods, imbalances in our neurotransmitters can leave us feeling impatient, so that we feel we don't have time to listen, even when we do.

Nichols believes that one key to listening is not to be emotionally reactive. He admits that such restraint can be difficult at times, but he emphasizes the importance of sitting down, listening to someone's grievances, and not responding until the other person has finished talking or is ready to hear your comments. When you do respond, it's important to acknowledge what the other person has said and to respond calmly. That doesn't mean you have to agree, but if you do disagree or even argue, you still maintain a sense of fair play.

Don't take everything personally. Celeste was an older woman and a careful driver who always followed the speed limit. One day, she came in to work upset because another driver had honked at her—not a little tap on the horn, but one of those long punitive honks. At work, Celeste also had a tendency to take other people's comments personally, as if she had said or done something wrong. She was a good worker, just as she was a good driver.

I explained to Celeste that a lot of what people say or do reflects more about their own personalities than it does about other people's behavior. Having driven with her, I knew she was a safe driver. I explained that impatient drivers might feel as if she was slowing them down, but their impatience wasn't her problem. It was theirs. Similarly, she could ignore the office blabbermouth because everyone felt that the person's gossip was annoying and simply to be tolerated.

. . .

In the next part of the book, I'll describe ways to improve specific mood and behavior problems, including anger, anxiety, depression, impatience, impulsiveness, irritability, mood swings, panic attacks, and obsessive-compulsive behavior.

PART III

Improving Your Specific Mood and Behavior Concerns

8

Dealing with Irritability, Anger, Aggressiveness, and Violent Behavior

In this part of the book, I organized much of my advice about nutrition, supplements, and lifestyle into specific plans for improving mood and behavior problems. These problems fall into several categories that include

- Irritability, pissy moods, anger, and physical violence
- Anxiety, nervousness, tension, fear, and panic
- Impulsive and distractible behavior
- Mood swings associated with fatigue, mental fuzziness, blood sugar problems, and being overweight
- Depression and down days
- Alcohol and drug abuse

Each grouping encompasses many related mood and behavior issues, ranging from mild to severe. For example, feelings of resentment are related to stronger feelings of anger and violent behavior. Similarly, anxiety ranges from vague feelings of nervousness to panic attacks. Sometimes minor mood problems escalate to more serious ones, and it's usually easier to correct these problems while they remain relatively minor. The chances of your physically hurting yourself or another person, or damaging your relationships, increase as your moods and behavior become more intense.

In these chapters, you'll notice that there is often overlap between moods. For example, anxiety is frequently intertwined with depression, and post-traumatic syndrome usually entails both anxiety and depression (although I have placed PTSD in the chapter addressing anxiety problems). I've categorized moods for the purpose of this book based on dominant characteristics.

Get Aware, Get Willing, and Get With It

One key step in improving moods and behavior is being proactive and fighting the inertia that often keeps us from changing our lives for the better. *Inertia* is a scientific term that describes an object's resistance to movement or its inability to stop moving once it's started. In this context, it refers to a person's resistance to change. Helen Selwitschka, R.N., a psychiatric nurse in Tucson, Arizona, sums up her anti-inertia strategy in a simple phrase: "Get aware, get willing, and get with it."

Although this maxim might sound like an oversimplification (along the lines of the "Just do it" advertising slogan), it actually lists steps that are necessary in the long-term effort to improve your moods, behavior, and quality of life. Don't let the long-term nature of the steps scare you off. You can begin working on all three steps almost immediately and simultaneously—even if you take only baby steps—and you'll quickly see the benefits. Selwitschka's view has been shaped by years of helping people with addictive and self-destructive moods and behavior patterns.

- First, you must become aware of your mood or behavior problem and how it affects your life and the people around you. This awareness may prompt you to seek professional psychological counseling and engage in personal introspection to understand what's wrong with your moods and behavior. At that point, you may realize that you would be happier if you improved some aspects of your life.

- Second, you must be willing to act on your newfound understanding and follow the recommendations of your counselor or therapist.

You will likely need to develop a plan or specific goals that describe what you will do differently.

- Third, you must be willing to act on your knowledge and your plan, working to modify your moods and your actions. Making these changes may be difficult, but with each baby step, you become more capable of making further changes. Those changes might include recognizing and changing bad behavior, modifying eating habits, taking nutritional supplements, and improving other aspects of your lifestyle.

Anger and Physical Violence

Feelings of anger encompass a wide range of negative and hostile feelings toward other people, as well as toward institutions (such as the government or political parties). Anger-related feelings and behavior (how you express your feelings of anger) include brooding, resentment, annoyance, aggravation, rudeness, sarcasm, passive-aggressiveness, impatience, irritability, inflammatory language, outbursts, negative energy, road rage, hatred, hostile-personality disorder, vital exhaustion, destructive behavior, juvenile delinquency, and adult criminal violence.

What You Should Know

Anger is a secondary emotion, meaning that it develops in response to a primary emotion, such as frustration, hurt, or pain. For example, if your spouse has a sexual affair, your feelings of hurt and betrayal may be expressed as anger. When you're angry with another person, give some thought to *why* you really feel angry—that is, the primary emotion triggering your anger. What has that person done to hurt or frustrate you?

People with hostile-personality disorder have a short fuse and react quickly and with intense anger to feelings of stress. This tendency toward explosive anger appears to stem from a combination of genetics and poor nutrition, resulting in low levels of certain neuronutrients and neurotransmitters. It's also a result of learned behavioral habits. The hair-trigger response that typifies hostile-personality disorder can be modified through dietary improvements, supplements, psychological counseling, and lifestyle changes.

Brooding and resentment are related to anger and, like a simmering dish, tend to cook. I'm sure you've heard the phrase "He's really stewing." Resentment is a feeling of anger that's bottled up. Often, resentment occurs when we feel slighted or put down, or feel that people are acting superior or trying to control us. People with feelings of resentment relive or brood about painful experiences, frequently thinking about what they would do differently if given the chance or what they might do to get even.

On a day-to-day basis, anger is expressed in many ways. Some people seem to be irritable, grumpy, cranky, or "on the warpath" most of the time, and they may take their anger out on people who had nothing to do with their original feelings of hurt. Chronically angry people also tend to misinterpret other people's words and actions and take them personally. Anger and resentment often feed their own escalation. For example, road rage usually results from pent-up frustration about traffic congestion, which may be expressed through horn honking, reckless speeding and lane changing, or freeway shootings. People who have angry outbursts are often described as losing it or having a meltdown.

Impatience is a form of annoyance and anger that's commonly seen in many people's driving habits. A person who is annoyed and impatient with traffic might tailgate, speed, and weave between lanes, only to be stopped at red lights, increasing his or her frustration, annoyance, and impatience. My father taught me the value of pacing while driving—that is, to time my speed so that I hit more green than red lights. This idea of pacing seems to be completely lost on many drivers. It is actually far less frustrating to drive a little slower but to hit more green lights.

Anger taps into primitive brain functions related to physical aggressiveness and survival. The epinephrine (adrenaline) release with anger increases our energy levels for a short while, an important survival trait. Alcohol, which reduces social inhibitions, often increases the expression of anger, either in words or physical actions. That's why alcohol is commonly associated with abusive behavior and fighting. For example, instances of "air rage" have typically involved airline passengers who get drunk and then verbally abuse or physically attack flight personnel.

Psychologists have long thought that anger is related to feelings of low self-esteem or self-worth; however, this idea is now being challenged. Some psychologists contend that poor self-esteem may, conversely, be the result of feelings of anger. There is evidence that anger is more related to a lack of control over one's life or an inability to change things for the better, often combined with a desire to get back at people who are believed to be responsible.

Is there anything good about anger? It's a normal emotion as long as it is appropriate to the situation and quickly dissipates afterward. Practicing forgiveness can help to reduce anger. Anger increases our physical energy and mental focus, which is good as long as the anger is not misplaced, misdirected, or hurtful.

Violent Behavior and Nutrition

Violent behavior is essentially a crescendo of anger. Over the last thirty-five years, a small number of researchers, law enforcement personnel, and psychiatrists have investigated how poor nutrition contributes to anger, destructive behavior, and violence. They have found that inadequate nutrition can alter moods, thinking processes, and a moral sense of what is right or wrong.

At the Pfeiffer Treatment Center, located in the Chicago suburb of Warrenville, doctors are researching the use of nutritional supplements to treat severe mood and behavioral disorders, including extreme anger, destructive behavior, and criminal violence. Staff at the center conduct a thorough nutritional and biochemical workup of patients and then prescribe a customized nutritional supplement regimen.

In an analysis of 207 randomly selected patients, the center's scientific director, William Walsh, Ph.D., found that customized supplements led to a 92 percent lower frequency of physical assaults and 53 percent fewer occurrences of property damage. Walsh reported that three-fourths of patients with intense angry outbursts and violent behavior had abnormally high levels of copper relative to zinc. In fact, the high-copper, low-zinc pattern is strongly associated with an explosive temper, "like a volcano going off." About one-third of the patients had difficulty dealing with sugar and other refined carbohydrates, which aggravated existing mood and behavior problems.

In his research, Walsh has consistently found nutrient-handling problems in violent criminals. In an analysis of mineral patterns in thirty serial killers and mass murderers, he frequently found elevated levels of lead or cadmium, which are highly toxic and interfere with normal brain chemistry. Walsh traced many of these mineral problems to low production of metallothionein, a sulfur-containing protein needed to properly use zinc and to protect against lead and cadmium.

In another study, C. Bernard Gesch, a professor of social work at Oxford University, England, tested the effects of a combination of supplements or placebos on 231 young adult prisoners eighteen years of age and older. The supplements were comparable to conventional once-a-day vitamin formulas, plus essential dietary fats (such as omega-3 fish oils and gamma-linolenic acid).

At the beginning of the study, almost all of the prisoners were found to be deficient in selenium, a mineral that can affect mood, and more than two-thirds of the prisoners were also deficient in magnesium, potassium, iodine, and zinc. Overall, prisoners taking the supplements for several months committed one-fourth fewer offenses. Similar benefits can be achieved in reducing less serious everyday mood and behavior problems.

> ## Quick Tip
>
> **Seven Fast Ways to Turn a Bad Mood Around**
> 1. Go to the bathroom. Don't laugh! It's a great place to hide out for a few minutes.
> 2. Rub your eyes (lightly, not enough to irritate them).
> 3. Wash your face.
> 4. Have a cup of green tea.
> 5. Go for a ten-minute walk as a time-out.
> 6. Eat a little protein, such as a couple of slices of deli turkey.
> 7. Lie on your back on the floor for five minutes and do some stretching exercises.

Psychological Tips for Dealing with Your Own Anger

You can cool down your own anger before it gets out of hand. Here are some ways.

Recognize that you're getting mad. Develop an internal tripwire to alert you to when your anger is building, instead of allowing it to flare up. Next, determine the specific trigger of your anger, such as something your boss or spouse said to you. Then, work on figuring out why you feel angry. Did someone insult you and catch you off guard, so that you couldn't think of a good response until later?

Cultivate your own reset switch. A reset switch is a lot like a circuit breaker that cuts off the electricity when there's a power surge. If you often find yourself becoming impatient or irritable, such as when traffic is moving too slow, use your emotional reset switch to improve your mood.

Take deep breaths. Simply taking three or four slow, deep breaths can change your brain chemistry and reduce your stress response, which is intertwined with feelings of anger. When stressed, people tend to take short, shallow breaths.

Practice visualization. Imagine yourself in a calmer situation. Follow my visualization guidelines in chapter 7.

Get it out physically but safely. It may help to physically release some of your anger, especially if you're a guy. A simple exercise is to clasp your hands together and push them against each other. Another is to squeeze a stress ball.

Develop a stronger physical release, if needed. Anger causes physical agitation, and you can reduce agitation through regular and intense physical activity in which you let loose without hurting anyone else. Try chopping wood or boxing with a punching bag in your house or a gym. Or create an area in your yard or basement where you can repeatedly kick a small garbage can, smash cans with a baseball bat, whack an inflatable dummy with your hands, or throw pillows or "clay pigeons" (See Quick Tip on page 174) against a wall. Just be careful to avoid accidentally hurting yourself or anyone else in the process.

Think realistically. If you're angry about slow traffic, ask yourself whether honking, speeding, running red lights, or weaving in and out of traffic will really save you much time. It won't save more than a minute; however, such driving habits may risk serious injury. Accept the fact that if traffic is congested, nothing you do will get you to your destination faster. (See the Serenity Prayer in chapter 2.) Being patient while driving will also lessen the chances of your inciting someone else's anger.

Talk about your feelings with someone you trust. Describing your frustration, hurt, or anger to a friend will release some of your feelings.

The experience is a lot like venting steam to reduce pressure in a pipe or a cooker. A close and understanding friend can help, as can a therapist.

Avoid situations that repeatedly trigger your anger. Certain situations are particularly trying, and it's best to avoid them if you can't find another solution. Consider the case of Peter, who was in a relationship with an emotionally demanding and petulant woman. They had serious arguments every few weeks, blaming each other for not doing the right thing. Counseling failed to help, so Peter ended the relationship. He realized that he felt less put upon and angry when he was by himself than when he was dating her.

Psychological Tips for Dealing with Someone Else's Anger

It can be tricky dealing with someone who is angry, especially if the anger is directed at you. Yet it can be done. Here are some ideas.

Don't engage the person. If someone honks at you, it might feel good to shout back or make an obscene gesture. Your actions may further fuel his anger, though, leading to a more aggressive and threatening response on his part.

Quick Tip

Heal Your Mind and Body . . . by Breaking Things?

We teach children not to intentionally break their toys or damage other property. Yet safely getting some of the anger out of your system can do a lot for your mental and physical health. The idea is a little like letting off steam to prevent an explosion.

On the grounds of the Bright Spot for Health, a nutritionally oriented medical clinic in Wichita, Kansas, stressed staff members and patients can walk over to a specified area to throw and break "clay pigeons." These are the same hardened clay disks used in sport target shooting. Of course, shooting isn't allowed here, so people can take a few clay disks, throw them against a wall, and enjoy seeing them shatter.

It works wonders. In one case, a patient with serious skin problems and a lot of repressed anger found that her skin tone improved within days of spending time tossing and breaking the clay disks.

Back off. Backing off involves consciously retreating, which is different from simply not engaging. This is especially important if you see body language that hints at impending violence. Calmly leave the immediate environment if another person is rapidly escalating his expression of anger (such as getting louder and louder and more physically agitated), throwing objects, verbally threatening to physically harm you, or trying to grab you. If you need an excuse—sometimes a very angry person may try to restrain you—say you've got to go to the bathroom. If there is violence, or if the angry person has a history of being violent, call 911.

Acknowledge the person's feelings. Don't argue with the angry person—doing so will likely escalate his expression of anger. Instead, listen and acknowledge his feelings, such as by saying, "I understand," or by rephrasing what he has said. This may have a calming effect because angry people often believe they are not being heard.

Speak softly and slowly. Speaking softly and slowly is usually non-threatening. Responding with a loud voice may be interpreted as arguing back. In addition, keep your comments short—speak in sentences, not long-winded paragraphs. People who are angry do not hear a lot.

Set your boundaries. If a person is mad at you and is being verbally abusive, set your boundaries firmly but politely. For example, if he calls you a name, calmly say that you'll listen so long as he sticks to the issues and doesn't call you names. If the verbal abuse continues, walk away without showing agitation.

Don't spread the anger. If Joe is mean to you, it might feel good to release your resentment and anger on Barbara, who just happens to be passing by. Anger can spread like an infection. If anger is directed at you, and you feel yourself getting angry, don't direct your anger at someone else.

Avoid abusive people. Abusive people may never touch you—they just slash you to pieces with their words and demands. Bosses can be especially abusive because of their own frustrations and their power over employees. Consider the case of John, whose boss regularly put him down to his face and in front of other people. John tried to transfer to another department in the company but eventually left for a new employer.

Sarcasm and Passive-Aggressive Behavior

Sarcasm and passive-aggressive behavior are two common expressions of anger. We often admire a person with a quick, sharp tongue, and sometimes we wish we could say things the way that person does. For example, the comedians Don Rickles and Joan Rivers excel in sarcasm. Yet sarcasm is as sharp as any dagger, and laughing at sarcasm is a little like laughing at someone who tortures kittens. It's a red flag.

Passive-aggressive behavior is another form of anger, although it is subtle and many people can be manipulated by it. Passive-aggressive people are angry because other people don't do what they would like. Instead of describing their feelings, though, they try to manipulate. They often act helpless and clingy, and they tend to be procrastinators. The passive-aggressive person is clever enough to look compliant or cooperative on the surface but may undermine projects with passive obstructionism or by making excuses. Passive-aggressive people may also be argumentative, which is intended to conceal their dependency. The behavior tends to alienate friends and coworkers, driving away the very people who might otherwise be supportive.

Vital Exhaustion—A Particular Type of Anger

Doctors have long understood that persistent feelings of anger are strongly associated with a higher risk of having a heart attack. Yet a condition known as vital exhaustion significantly increases the risk of a heart attack. Vital exhaustion is characterized by a combination of three feelings: extreme fatigue and lack of energy, increasing irritability and anger, and a sense of demoralization.

Psychologically, irritability and anger stem from frustration with feeling beaten down in life and being overwhelmingly tired. The anger may be expressed as flailing about and being irritated at people. Individuals with vital exhaustion are stressed and have high levels of the hormone cortisol. Yet evidence also points to poor eating habits as a contributing factor. People with fat around the middle (belly fat) and prediabetes are more likely to suffer from vital exhaustion. In fact, the larger a person's belly, the more likely that he or she will develop vital exhaustion.

People are more likely to feel fatigued if they don't eat regular meals and they tend to consume junk foods, such as soft drinks, sweets, and fast foods. To increase energy levels, reduce or eliminate these foods from your diet and eat more protein. Simply eating a couple of slices of deli turkey will improve your energy level and mood.

Dealing with Premenstrual Irritability

People often debate whether premenstrual syndrome (PMS) is an actual medical condition or just a natural part of a woman's life. The truth is that mild PMS symptoms affect upward of 90 percent of menstruating women, and an estimated 8 to 20 percent women experience severe symptoms. Physical symptoms include abdominal and back pain, migraines, and other types of headaches. Behavioral symptoms include irritability, a "climbing-the-walls" feeling, and mood swings.

There is an obvious biological underpinning to PMS symptoms, and some women are far more susceptible to shifting hormone levels because of genetics or nutrition. Certain nutrients, such as the B-complex vitamins, influence the liver's ability to process and break down hormones, and nutritional deficiencies and imbalances can contribute to prolonged elevated estrogen levels.

B-complex supplements have been found to calm women's moods, and vitamin B6 may be particularly important. It's also a mild diuretic, reducing uncomfortable premenstrual puffiness. Many other nutrients have been found helpful in lessening PMS symptoms, most likely because they correct deficiencies. In one study, described in the *Archives of Internal Medicine*, women consuming ample amounts of vitamin D (700 IU daily) were 41 percent less likely to have PMS symptoms. Similarly, a high intake of calcium (1,200 mg daily) was associated with a 30 percent lower risk of PMS symptoms.

In a separate study, British researchers reported that the herb St. John's wort significantly reduced PMS symptoms. The researchers found that a standardized St. John's wort supplement, 300 mg taken three times daily, cut overall PMS symptoms by half and that two-thirds of the women in the study benefited from the herb.

St. John's wort improves the liver's ability to break down chemicals, including hormones. It also contains many beneficial antioxidants, which may decrease pain and improve mood; however, the herb may diminish the effectiveness of oral contraceptives.

Eating Habits

To temper your feelings of anger, follow my dietary recommendations in chapter 5 and emphasize high-quality proteins, such as chicken, turkey, and fish, as well as abundant high-fiber vegetables. The protein provides amino acids that are needed to make neurotransmitters, and both the protein and the vegetable fiber help to stabilize blood sugar levels. Stable blood sugar levels will reduce the risk of mood swings.

Avoid soft drinks sweetened with sugar, high-fructose corn syrup, and other types of sugar (including "natural" sugars). In addition, stay away from deep-fried foods such as fried chicken and French fries. You will likely benefit from reducing your intake of caffeine (coffee and colas), energy drinks, and alcohol. If you have trouble giving up coffee, limit your intake to two cups in the morning and don't add sugar. As an alternative to sugar, consider the herbal sweetener stevia, which is available in health food stores.

If you often have to work for long stretches and don't have time for a nutritious lunch or dinner, keep some healthful snacks handy. These snacks might include slices of deli meats (chicken, turkey, beef, or ham), deli cheese (as long as you are not allergic to dairy products), or nuts (unsalted peanuts, cashews, pecans, or almonds). It won't take more than a minute to eat some of these foods. You might keep a can of tuna or sardines or a couple of apples handy as well.

Helpful Supplements

Many different supplements can mellow your mood. Most will generally help within a few days, and some within an hour or two. Ideally, you should work with a nutritionally oriented physician or psychiatrist who can order blood tests and identify specific deficiencies. If you are trying to improve your moods on your own, try the following supplements.

Multivitamin. As part of your nutritional foundation, take a high-potency multivitamin supplement, along the lines of what I described in chapter 4. It should contain at least 50 mg each of the major B vitamins, including B1, B2, B3, and B6. Formulations will vary somewhat, and larger amounts of vitamins B3 and B6 are fine. Studies have found that multivitamins can help to reduce mood swings, aggressive behavior, and explosive rage. Note: Vitamin B2 will turn your urine bright yellow. The yellow color is normal and not harmful.

Vitamin C. The first symptoms of low vitamin C intake are irritability and fatigue, both of which are usually present with anger. Brain levels of vitamin C are significantly higher than levels in the blood. Vitamin C is needed to make certain neurotransmitters, and it protects the brain from amphetamines—one clue to its mind-calming benefits. Vitamin C is also necessary to make carnitine, a compound involved in burning fats for energy in brain and all other cells.

Omega-3 fish oils. These contain eicosapentaenoic acid (EPA) and docosahexaenoic acid (DHA). Several studies have found that low intakes of these essential dietary fats are related to violence and murder. Not surprisingly, these nutrients have been found particularly useful in reducing aggressive and hostile behavior, including aggressive driving, bullying, verbal abusiveness, and fighting. The omega-3s are incorporated into cell membranes (walls), where they help brain cells to communicate with one another. They also dampen an overactive immune system, which seems to play a role in mood disorders. Start with 3 grams of fish oils daily; you can safely increase the dose up to 10 grams daily. *Note*: The omega-3 fish oils have a mild blood-thinning effect. Alternatively, you may try 1.5 grams daily of DHA.

Magnesium. If you have persistent feelings of irritability, take 400 mg of magnesium citrate, which is better absorbed than other forms of magnesium. Magnesium is a muscle relaxant and a cofactor in the production of serotonin. *Note*: If a single dose of 400 mg loosens your stools, take 200 mg twice daily.

GABA and L-theanine. Daily supplements of GABA (gamma aminobutyric acid) and L-theanine can increase the brain's alpha waves, which are associated with relaxation. A particularly good product is called

"200 mg of Zen," made by Allergy Research Group. The recommended dose of two capsules, which can be taken once or twice daily, provides 500 mg of GABA and 200 mg of L-theanine. A similar product from the Nutricology label of the same company provides 275 mg of GABA and 100 mg of L-theanine. (See the appendix for ordering information.) You can buy other brands of L-theanine, but look for the "SunTheanine" logo on the label, a sign of quality.

Mellow Mood. This proprietary supplement contains GABA, the SunTheanine brand of L-theanine, B vitamins, magnesium, and vitamin C. Taken regularly, it can take the edge off bad moods. If you want to take just one supplement to keep things as simple as possible, I highly recommend Mellow Mood. It's available from Carlson Laboratories (800-323-4141 or www.carlsonlabs.com).

5-HTP. If you have difficulty sleeping, take 50 mg of 5-HTP (5-hydroxy-tryptophan) about one hour before bed. This supplement is the immediate precursor to serotonin, and it may reduce aggression. If you notice some benefits from 5-HTP, but not as much as you would like, increase the dosage to 100 mg before bed. If you continue to feel tense or edgy during the day, take 50 to 100 mg three times daily: 15 minutes before breakfast or at least one hour away from eating any food. You can purchase a high-quality 5-HTP product from Carlson Laboratories and Thorne Research. (See the appendix for ordering information.)

Note: If you are taking any medications, such as antidepressants, for psychiatric or neurological disorders, you may start to feel overmedicated after taking supplements. As you use natural substances to improve your neuronutrients, you will need less of your medications. Please work with your physician to adjust your medications during this transition period.

Lifestyle Recommendations

If you are irritable, feel angry, have explosive outbursts, or have a tendency toward destructive behavior (breaking or damaging objects) or violence (threatening or actually hurting another person), you can take several steps to turn down the volume.

Seek professional counseling. Intense or persistent anger is potentially dangerous to you and other people. Your anger may also be a sign of depression (see chapter 12). Counseling, which is a form of talk therapy, may help you understand the social situations and your own behavior patterns that lead to feelings of irritability and anger. Talk therapy would be best if it were done in tandem with nutritional therapies. Talking with trusted friends may have some benefits, but a good counselor will guide you to your own insights instead of simply offering solutions.

Avoid people or situations that trigger your anger. Shielding yourself against anger triggers is a good interim step. For example, if a particular person gets under your skin, do your best to avoid or minimize your time with that person. If certain situations generate a lot of stress and

How Hank Learned to Lighten Up

Hank worked with customers at an automobile service center. It was important for him to leave work by 5:30 p.m. After all, he had already put in a long day by that time. A couple times a week, however, customers came in around 5:20 to pay for their service, get an explanation of the work that was done, and pick up their cars.

When this happened, Hank had to stay until at least 5:45. He was irritated, often visibly, and sometimes made critical comments to late-arriving customers. Ronald, Hank's boss, saw that the customers didn't like Hank's attitude, but he also respected Hank's knowledge and how well he usually performed his work.

One day Ronald discussed the situation with Hank, who later described the conversation to his wife. Hank's wife suggested that he take an anti-stress B-complex vitamin supplement and also talk with a counselor. The counselor suggested that Hank adjust his expectations, that he think more in terms of working until 5:45, and that he also negotiate for some time off to compensate.

After talking with his boss, Hank got a little comp time in the form of an occasional extra half-hour for lunch. The change in expectations and sometimes having extra time off helped Hank to feel better about working longer. The B vitamins seemed to mellow him out overall, and customers soon commented on his positive attitude.

make you angry, avoid those situations. Eventually, however, you should be able to face these situations or people without reacting to them.

Increase your brain's alpha waves. You can reduce feelings of irritation and anger by boosting your brain's alpha waves, which are a type of brain wave associated with relaxation. Meditation and yoga are well known for boosting alpha waves. So is drinking green tea. Part of the effect of green tea is related to its high content of L-theanine, but even the act of sitting and sipping tea is relaxing. (In contrast, coffee drinkers often feed a caffeine addiction or use the beverage as a stimulant.)

Slow, methodical activities, such as sweeping the floor, cleaning, or baking, can also be relaxing, insightful, meditative experiences. To turn mundane activities into meditative experiences, it helps to be in the moment (as I discussed in chapter 7) and pay attention to the details of what you're doing, instead of simply rushing through the activity. Many companies sell tapes and CDs designed to heighten certain mental states, including the production of alpha waves. One of the best of these companies is the Monroe Institute. (See the appendix for ordering information.)

9

Reducing Anxiety, Panic Attacks, and Obsessive-Compulsive Behavior

Our modern societies generate a never-ending stream of anxiety, with constant work pressures, responsibilities and chores at home, job-security worries, concerns about health and finances, argumentative talk radio, and fears of terrorism, to name but a few sources. This anxiety contributes to our feeling stressed out and is made worse by the consumption of coffee and sugar, stimulants that increase our edgy feelings and, ultimately, our physical fatigue.

For many people, feelings of stress and anxiety peak between Thanksgiving and Christmas because of family and shopping pressures, long lines in stores, and traffic jams (combined with dietary lapses). The result is that the Christmas season brings out the worst in our behavior—irritability, rudeness, and pushiness—not the cherished qualities of giving and tolerance.

In this chapter, I describe a variety of anxiety-related mood and behavior problems, as well as nutrition and lifestyle changes to lessen them.

Feelings of Anxiety, Panic, and Obsessive-Compulsiveness

Feelings of anxiety range from simple nervousness to being stressed out, to sudden and overwhelming panic attacks. We express the type and intensity of anxiety with a variety of words, including impatience, tension, jumpiness, agitation, nervousness, worry, apprehension, dread, fear, and panic. High-strung and jittery people are typically so anxious that they seem like stretched-out rubber bands that are about to snap. The now-antiquated term *nervous breakdown* referred to physical and mental exhaustion after prolonged, intense anxiety. Furthermore, when we're anxious, random thoughts and worries seem to enter our mind and we may have trouble getting rid of them, which in some people contributes to obsessive-compulsive behavior.

What You Should Know

It's normal to occasionally have situation-dependent anxieties and jitters, such as when we're on a first date, on a job interview, or speaking in front of a group. Anxieties become problematic when they are chronic and they interfere with normal daily activities and relationships with other people. Of special concern are two types of anxieties: those that develop without specific, recognizable, or rational causes; and mild or occasional feelings of anxiety that intensify into either acute or chronic feelings.

Anxieties take a toll on our physical health. They are driven by stress, and they also fuel feelings of stress. When you're anxious, your body's levels of the stress hormone cortisol remain high, with long-term physical and mental consequences. Chronically high cortisol levels kill off brain cells.

An estimated 19 million people in the United States are affected by anxiety disorders; this statistic generally reflects cases identified by health care professionals, such as counselors and doctors. The more fuzzy or anonymous anxieties—those without obvious causes—tend to fall under the medical radar. The most common signs of these anxieties are tension, irritability, and worry—all rampant in today's stress-filled lifestyles.

Phobias, such as a fear of heights or spiders, are probably the most prevalent form of anxiety and, for many people, are relatively innocuous. Mild phobias (such as a fear of heights) are little more than personality quirks. People who have them typically avoid anxiety-triggering exposures or quickly retreat from them; however, more severe phobias that interfere with day-to-day activities warrant professional treatment.

Some research has found that abdominal obesity—belly fat—is strongly associated with feelings of anxiety. The specific relationship between obesity and anxiety is not entirely clear, but it's likely that the poor eating habits that cause obesity also result in a deficiency of neuronutrients.

General Feelings

When you're anxious, you worry about big and little things, everything and anything, nearly all of the time, and you can't shake your concerns. Some people call you a worrywart. You may be jumpy, jittery, or impatient, or switch rapidly between many different activities at work, at home, or in the car. You may be irritable because no one else seems to do things the "right way" or fast enough to suit you. Your breathing is often tight and shallow, you have difficulty relaxing, and you can't get a good night's sleep because you fret so much.

Many people experience this low-grade but persistent level of anxiety, which is not easily noticed during cursory medical exams. This anxiety results from feelings of being stressed, although the stress can just as easily come from within a person. The anxiety doesn't disappear after work or chores are completed.

Some people multitask in order to get jobs done and reduce anxiety, but multitasking often fuels anxiety instead of relieving it. Multitasking prevents the mind from clearly focusing on individual tasks; the mind is so anxious that it jumps from one task to the next. Because the mind is not focused, anxiety may trigger impulsive and rash actions. I'll come back to this in the next chapter when I discuss impulsive and distractible behavior.

As with stress, anxiety often derails eating habits. When you feel worried, you might forget to eat until your blood sugar level falls and your stomach aches. At that point, the fastest food is fast food—not the type of nourishment that supports your neuronutrients and good-mood neurotransmitters.

The medical term for sustained and relatively intense feelings of anxiety is *generalized anxiety disorder*. It's characterized by experiencing excessive worry (defined as "apprehensive expectation") and anxiety on most days over a six-month period. Generalized anxiety disorder is commonly associated with physical symptoms, such as fatigue, restlessness, heart palpitations, and dizziness.

Psychological Tips

It's important to adopt behavioral changes that reduce stress and anxiety and also to block anxious feelings when you feel them increasing. Here are some tips. Refer back to chapter 7 for more suggestions.

- First and foremost, if certain people or situations trigger your anxiety, avoid your exposure to them—at least, until you are better able to control your anxiety. If a stressful situation develops unexpectedly, try to calmly remove yourself from it.

- Take three or four slow, deep breaths.

- Make a cup of hot green tea and sip it slowly.

- Lie on the floor and do some stretching exercises with your arms and legs for five minutes.

- If you have a pet, spend a few minutes petting and talking to it.

- Visualize (or daydream for a few minutes about) a calmer, more relaxing place, such as the beach or a forest.

Eating Habits

We ply ourselves with stimulants to help us wake up in the morning and to keep us going during the day, and these same stimulants can cause edgy feelings. In light of that, my dietary recommendations are straightforward: greatly reduce or avoid all caffeine, eliminate sugars and refined carbohydrates, and eat more protein, healthy fats, and high-fiber nonstarchy vegetables.

Drinking too many caffeine beverages increases our jittery, anxious feelings. One way it does this is by raising levels of lactate in the body, which promotes anxiety. Vitamin B3 enhances the breakdown of lactate.

One or two cups of coffee a day are not a problem for most people. Yet five to ten cups daily can be, as can fewer cups of a high-caffeine brew, such as Starbucks. Starbucks' beverages contain extremely large amounts of caffeine. A twelve-ounce cup of Starbucks coffee has 195 mg of caffeine, or a little more than 16 mg per ounce. Even high-caffeine energy drinks, such as Red Bull, SoBe No Fear, Full Throttle, Monster, and Mountain Dew MDX, have less caffeine than Starbucks' coffee. Regular Mountain Dew and cola soft drinks also have appreciable amounts of caffeine, as well as sugars or the artificial sweetener aspartame (which is closely related to the stimulating neurotransmitter phenylethylamine).

If you are a regular coffee drinker, you know that caffeine can be as addictive as alcohol or street drugs. Missing a cup of coffee—not getting your hit—can give you a headache or leave you feeling exhausted. Just as too much coffee can make you edgy, so can missing a cup. Coffee withdrawal symptoms usually disappear after a few days, though.

Green tea, which can be consumed hot or as iced tea, may be a suitable coffee substitute. Although green tea contains caffeine, it also has large amounts of L-theanine, which can offset the effect of caffeine. Some people are so caffeine-sensitive, however, that even green tea can produce a jittery feeling and restless sleep.

Fatigue is frequently intertwined with anxiety and caffeine consumption. We are more likely to be irritable when we're tired. Excessive caffeine consumption interferes with sleep, and caffeine addicts commonly wake up feeling tired. To become more alert, they repeat the cycle by drinking more caffeinated beverages and eating sugary foods. Similarly, sugary foods and refined carbohydrates play havoc with blood sugar levels, increasing mental fuzziness and tiredness. This often prompts people to consume more caffeine and sugary foods.

In contrast, high-quality proteins (such as chicken, turkey, and fish) and nonstarchy vegetables (such as salads with oil and vinegar dressing) tend to stabilize blood sugar levels. Eating an egg, some deli meat, or leftover meat from an earlier meal for breakfast can help you to maintain energy for hours.

Although I generally recommend lean proteins, some research indicates that a moderately high-fat diet can reduce anxiety. When researchers fed healthy men high-fat diets (with 41 percent of the calories coming from fat), the subjects' anxiety and tension levels decreased. Men eating low-fat diets had no improvement in moods. The high-fat diet contained saturated fat but also ample amounts of more healthful monounsaturated and polyunsaturated fats.

Helpful Supplements

Most anxiety disorders have common biochemical features, but they differ in intensity. Because of this, many of the same supplements are useful for these disorders but in different dosages.

B-complex vitamins. A high-potency B-complex (or a high-potency multivitamin) is the most important supplement for reducing anxiety. A supplement containing 25 to 50 mg of vitamins B1, B2, and B3 should contain relative amounts of other B vitamins. Consider adding an additional 100 mg of vitamin B6 to enhance your production of serotonin, a relaxing neurotransmitter. If your diet has tended to be high in sugars and carbohydrates (e.g., pasta or bread), add 100 mg of additional vitamin B1. *Note*: Take B vitamins in the morning or the early afternoon, with food. Large amounts of vitamin B6 may overstimulate dream activity, leading to restless sleep.

Vitamin C. The first symptoms of inadequate vitamin C intake are irritability and fatigue, both of which are commonly associated with anxiety. Vitamin C helps to prevent brain toxicity from stimulants. Although supplemental vitamin C by itself is unlikely to have a dramatic effect on mood, it is extremely important. Take 1,000 to 4,000 mg daily, divided into three or four daily dosages, with or without food. *Note*: If you develop loose stools, reduce the dosage.

Magnesium. Muscle tenseness is a sign of stress and anxiety, and the body needs magnesium for muscle relaxation. Muscle spasms (charley horses) likely indicate inadequate magnesium levels. Many people consume too much calcium (from dairy foods and supplements) and not enough magnesium. Take 400 mg daily of magnesium citrate or magnesium citrate malate, with meals. If you develop loose stools, divide the dosage so that you take it twice daily, or reduce it slightly. Some people may also benefit from calcium supplements. Try 300 mg daily of calcium citrate, combined with 800 IU of vitamin D (to enhance the absorption of calcium).

L-theanine. This amino acid (protein building block) increases the brain's production of GABA (gamma aminobutyric acid) and relaxing alpha waves. It can take the edge off anxiety, often within thirty to forty minutes. Take 200 mg of GABA one to three times daily, at least one hour away from eating food. Many companies sell L-theanine, but look for the "SunTheanine" logo on the bottle, which indicates a high-quality source.

Mellow Mood. This proprietary supplement contains GABA, the SunTheanine brand of L-theanine, B vitamins, magnesium, and vitamin C. The ingredients help reduce anxiety and improve mental focus. Mellow Mood is perfect if you don't want to hassle with a lot of supplements. It's available from Carlson Laboratories (800-323-4141 or www.carlsonlabs.com).

Lactium. This relatively new supplement contains a peptide (similar to a protein) that is naturally found in dairy products. Studies have found that supplemental Lactium can reduce stress-induced anxiety. Take 200 mg in the morning and again in the evening, or follow the label directions for use.

Gamma linolenic acid (GLA). Researchers found that supplements of borage oil, providing 1.3 grams of GLA, help you to become less sensitive to stress. The mechanism is unclear. GLA is an anti-inflammatory dietary fat, however, and stress triggers a heightened inflammatory reaction. Take 1 to 3 grams daily.

Melatonin. If your anxiety levels make it difficult to sleep, take melatonin one to two hours before bedtime. Be sure you are at home when you take it the first time because it may make you drowsy. Melatonin is a hormone made by the pineal gland, and supplements contain a synthetic version of it (so you don't have to worry about contracting a disease from animal-brain products). Normally, the body's levels increase in the evening and induce a sleepy feeling, but stress, stimulants, artificial light, and excessive time indoors disrupt its production. Some people need a very small amount of melatonin to achieve the desired effect, whereas others require much more. Take 0.25 or 0.5 mg to start (you may have to split a tablet to get this small dose), one to two hours before bedtime. If it has no effect, increase the amount by about 1 mg, up to a maximum of 9 mg, on each subsequent evening until it helps. Don't take more than 9 mg of melatonin a day.

Valerian. Valerian (*Valeriana officinalis*) is a sedative herb that's especially helpful if you have trouble sleeping. It was used by Hippocrates, the father of medicine, 2,500 years ago and has remained a popular therapeutic herb in Europe. Studies found that it helps to promote restful sleep. When using valerian, follow label directions because the forms (tablets, capsules, tinctures) provide different potencies. *Note*: Be cautious using valerian with any other sedative herb (such as kava), with melatonin, or with tranquilizers (such as Valium) and sleeping pills. Check with a medical doctor or a naturopathic physician before combining any of these sedatives.

Chamomile. Chamomile (also known as *German chamomile, Matricaria chamomilla, Matricaria recutita,* and *Chamomilla recutita*) was used by ancient Egyptians, Greeks, and Romans to treat a variety of ills, including upset stomach and skin problems. It also has anxiety-reducing and mild sedative benefits. If you take it in capsule or tablet form, follow the label directions because potencies vary among manufacturers. Chamomile has a light apple smell and a grassy taste, and it makes a tasty hot tea, especially with the addition of a little honey. *Note*: Chamomile is related to ragweed, and some people with ragweed allergies may be sensitive to the herb.

Lifestyle Recommendations

How can you counter the stresses of modern life? In a few words, take more deep breaths and slow down. Anxiety often develops as a form of nervousness related to having too much to do and not having enough time. Follow my advice in chapter 7 to create more time and add balance in your life. As so many other authors have advised over the years, ignore the small, inconsequential stuff.

- Give yourself enough time for work and home duties. You'll most likely have to schedule your activities, work from lists, and ignore less essential pursuits.

- Resist the temptation to multitask. It is far more relaxing—and efficient—to focus on one task at a time. Use other activities as breaks to refresh your mind.

- Take the time to prepare your food without feeling rushed. Use fresh and wholesome ingredients, not packaged foods intended for microwave heating.

- Whether you eat at home or in restaurants, eat slowly and chew your food. Doing so will reinforce your other anxiety-reducing activities, and you'll also enjoy the taste of your food more.

Anxiety Attacks, Panic Attacks, and Panic Disorder

Extreme episodes of anxiety and panic attacks are the most intense and scary forms of anxiety. I once had a neighbor, Dave, a Vietnam War veteran, who was unable to work because of wounds he had suffered in combat. Dave invited a number of people, including me, to attend a July 4 fireworks display at a nearby military base. I had wondered whether he might find the sound of fireworks reminiscent of his battlefield experiences, and my concern was justified. Dave became unnerved and anxious by the loud explosionlike sounds and the flashing lights of the fireworks. His breathing became labored, and he was a little shaken by the experience, but he was still able to drive us home. Dave had suffered an anxiety attack.

Panic attacks are far more overwhelming than what Dave had experienced. They are episodes of anxiety that increase suddenly in intensity, usually for no apparent reason, and lead to an overwhelming sense of terror or fear of death. It's almost as if the brain overloads and short-circuits. Symptoms include shortness of breath, heart palpitations, chest pain, and a fear of going crazy or losing control. Often, the person having a panic attack feels as if he or she is having a heart attack. Perhaps not surprisingly, people with a history of panic attacks have almost twice the risk of developing heart disease.

An estimated 2.4 million people in the United States experience panic attacks each year, and many celebrities have publicly acknowledged that they have experienced panic attacks, including Barbra Streisand, Anthony Hopkins, Eric Clapton, Kim Basinger, Nicole Kidman, and Oprah Winfrey. Well-known historical figures, including Abraham Lincoln, Edvard Munch (painter of *The Scream*), Sigmund Freud, and Sir Isaac Newton, had them as well.

The country-western singer Naomi Judd has often talked about her panic attacks in magazine and television interviews. After Judd was diagnosed with a hepatitis C infection in the early 1990s, she began to have totally disabling panic attacks that kept her from performing on stage. In an interview with Larry King on CNN, Judd described a panic attack as an "intense, absolutely senseless fear" that was almost like having a hallucination. Over several years, she was able to overcome both her hepatitis C infection and her panic attacks through a combination of faith, humor, managing stress, spending time in nature, taking vitamin supplements, and exercising.

After the first panic attack, a person may feel subsequent attacks start to build to a crescendo. When a person repeatedly experiences panic attacks, he or she is diagnosed as having panic disorder. Some people become so petrified of experiencing more panic attacks that they physically isolate themselves, staying home and avoiding people and unfamiliar situations.

Psychological Tips

When you sense the early signs of a panic attack, find a private place (such as your home, an office with a door you can close, or your parked car) to isolate yourself from stimuli. Close your eyes and begin to breathe deeply. If you can lie back, do so. Visualize yourself in the most peaceful setting you can imagine, such as in bed on a Sunday morning or stretched out near a quiet pond.

Whether you can isolate yourself or you are in a crowd of people, it's important to feel grounded. You can do this by pressing the palm of your hand against a heavy, solid object, such as a wall or a desk. Strange as it might seem, touching a massive object can help you to feel less anxious and panicky.

Eating Habits

People suffering from panic attacks should strive to stabilize their eating habits and blood sugar with regular meals. Bouts of low blood sugar may precipitate or aggravate panic attacks. That's because hypoglycemia can lead to physical symptoms that include shakiness and unsteadiness. Therefore, it is paramount that you avoid sugary foods (such as candies, doughnuts, and pastries) and refined carbohydrates (including bread, pasta, and pizza). Do not consume deep-fried foods, such as fried chicken or French fries, because they interfere with the body's use of omega-3 fats and gamma-linolenic acid.

Your diet should emphasize nutrient-dense food. Build meals around healthful protein sources, such as fish, chicken, and turkey. Fish is particularly important because it is rich in mood-enhancing omega-3 fats. Also include ample amounts of nonstarchy, high-fiber vegetables, such as steamed green beans, broccoli, and cauliflower, as well as salad greens. Small amounts of brown, red, purple, or black rice are fine, as is an occasional baked yam or sweet potato.

Large amounts of caffeine can cause symptoms similar to those that occur in the early stages of a panic attack, so you should wean yourself from caffeine. Sometimes, people with panic disorder cannot distinguish between symptoms of excessive caffeine intake and those of a panic attack. Fear of a panic attack can actually accelerate the onset of symptoms.

In certain cases, irritable bowel syndrome (IBS) is associated with panic attacks. Some researchers believe that's because IBS can be so embarrassing. There may be another explanation, however; 95 percent of the body's serotonin is made in the gut. A lack of serotonin production might make the digestive tract irritable, just as it can make the mind jumpy.

Helpful Supplements

B-complex vitamins. Take a high-potency B-complex (or a high-potency multivitamin) containing 50 to 75 mg of vitamins B1, B2, and B3 and relative amounts of other B vitamins. Consider adding an additional 100 mg of the more biologically active form of vitamin B6, called pyridoxyl-5-phosphate, as well as an additional 500 mg of vitamin B3 (niacinamide). *Note*: Take B vitamins in the morning or the early afternoon, with food—not in the evening.

Inositol. Functionally related to B vitamins, inositol has been shown to significantly diminish the occurrence of panic attacks. This is noteworthy because only 70 percent of patients with panic attacks respond to conventional medical therapies. In one study, researchers reported that 18 grams of inositol daily for one month reduced the number of panic attacks from six or seven weekly to only two or three. In a separate study, researchers found that 12 grams of inositol daily lessened the frequency and the severity of panic attacks, as well as the severity of associated agoraphobia (fear of public places). The number of panic attacks declined from an average of ten per week to about three and one-half after one month of supplementation.

By itself, inositol supplementation is more effective than pharmaceutical treatments; however, 12 to 18 grams daily translates to a lot of capsules or tablets. You can cut down on the number of pills by getting a prescription for inositol from your physician and having it filled by a compounding (custom) pharmacy. You might also be able to take less inositol (in the range of 4 to 6 grams daily) by combining it with a high-potency B-complex supplement and 5-HTP. On occasion, inositol will increase symptoms, in which case you should try one of the other recommended supplements.

Niacinamide. Extra amounts of this form of vitamin B3 might be helpful in alleviating anxiety, particularly when combined with the B-complex vitamins and 5-HTP. Try 1,000 mg twice daily. *Note*: Although the niacin form of vitamin B3 causes an intense flush, niacinamide does not.

Magnesium. A mild deficiency of magnesium has been associated with anxiety. In addition, a lack of magnesium increases blood levels of lactate, which is associated with anxiety. Take 400 to 600 mg daily of magnesium citrate or magnesium citrate malate, in divided doses with meals. If you develop loose stools, decrease the dose slightly.

GABA and L-theanine. Gamma aminobutyric acid is one of the body's key relaxing neurotransmitters. Take 500 mg one to three times daily, at least one hour prior to eating food. Consider combining it with L-theanine, which boosts the body's production of GABA. Take 200 mg of L-theanine one to three times daily with GABA.

Mellow Mood. Again, this proprietary supplement contains GABA, the SunTheanine brand of L-theanine, B vitamins, magnesium, and vitamin C—all substances that help the mind settle down. It's available from Carlson Laboratories (800-323-4141 or www.carlsonlabs.com).

Lactium. This supplement contains a natural dairy-derived peptide (like a protein) that may ease feelings of panic and panic attacks. Take 400 mg in the morning and again in the evening, or follow the label directions for use.

5-HTP. This supplement, 5-hydroxytryptophan, is the immediate pre-cursor to serotonin, the calming neurotransmitter that most psychotropic prescription drugs aim to elevate. Take 50 mg one to three times daily, apart from meals. If you can purchase tryptophan, it has the advantage

Quick Tip

How to Avoid Serotonin Syndrome

Serotonin syndrome is a serious medical condition caused by excessive levels of the neurotransmitter. It can develop when a person takes too much of a serotonin-enhancing drug or too many serotonin-boosting drugs.

Although serotonin syndrome can result in death, most cases are mild and are characterized by confusion, agitation, manic behavior, and anxiety. The syndrome can also cause rapid heartbeat, high or low blood pressure, tremors, and nausea.

Serotonin syndrome was rare before the 1960s. Its incidence began to increase with the widespread use of monoamine oxidase (MAO) inhibitor drugs for treating depression. The risk of serotonin syndrome has continued to grow with the wide use of selective serotonin reuptake inhibitor (SSRI) drugs, such as Prozac and Zoloft, which are designed to maintain high serotonin levels.

Usually, the risk of serotonin syndrome becomes greater when a person takes two medications (including L-tryptophan and 5-HTP) that boost serotonin levels through different mechanisms. For this reason, it's wise to work with a health care professional if you want to segue from a drug to a natural treatment.

of being more versatile biochemically. The dosage for tryptophan is higher, 500 mg one to three times daily, at least one hour before or after eating.

Post-Traumatic Stress Disorder

Post-traumatic stress disorder (PTSD) is an anxiety disorder that may affect 30 percent or more of all soldiers who have experienced combat. Other people who have experienced or witnessed traumatic events, including child abuse, criminal assaults such as rape, terrorist acts, automobile accidents, and airplane crashes, may also suffer from PTSD. The symptoms include anxiety, which is often intertwined with depression, as well as a tendency to be easily startled, have flashbacks and nightmares, be sensitive to noise, be hypervigilant, feel emotionally numbed, or have panic attacks.

Psychological Tips

Post-traumatic stress disorder is serious. The earlier it is treated, however, the quicker a person's recovery is likely to be. Treatment should include psychological counseling (talk therapy), nutrition, supplements, and medications when appropriate. Counseling may entail exposure therapy to relive the experience and to dull the response to memories of it.

As a general rule, people with or recovering from PTSD do better in less stressful work and home environments, insulated from loud or steady background noises, and with consistent emotional support from family and friends.

Eating Habits

Though often ignored, a wholesome and nutritious diet should be a fundamental part of any PTSD recovery program. First, healthy foods provide needed neuronutrients. Second, preparing such foods can be a relaxing and meditative experience. Third, eating them in a calm setting can help to lessen feelings of stress and anxiety.

Strictly limit your intake of sugars and carbohydrates, which reduce your body's levels of vitamin B1. Adhere to the dietary guidelines in chapter 5.

Helpful Supplements

Because of the severity of PTSD, it would be best for you to obtain a full nutritional workup, including blood chemistry and dietary analysis, from a physician. (See the appendix.) If this is not possible, try the following supplements in the order they're described. These supplements will likely reduce both anxiety and depression. Give each supplement two weeks to determine whether it is helping.

B-complex vitamins. Take a high-potency B-complex (or a high-potency multivitamin) containing 50 mg of vitamins B1, B2, and B3 and relative amounts of other B vitamins. Consider adding an additional 100 mg of vitamin B6 to enhance your production of serotonin, a relaxing neurotransmitter. If your diet has tended to be high in sugars and refined carbohydrates, take an additional 100 mg of vitamin B1. *Note*: Take B vitamins in the morning or the early afternoon, with food. Large amounts of vitamin B6 may overstimulate dream activity, leading to restless sleep.

Vitamin C. Vitamin C will alleviate feelings of fatigue and irritability. Take 1,000 to 4,000 mg of vitamin C daily, divided into three or four daily dosages, with or without food. *Note*: If you develop loose stools, decrease the dosage.

Magnesium. If you feel as if your muscles are tense and you have difficulty unwinding, add magnesium supplements. Take 400 mg daily of magnesium citrate or magnesium citrate malate, with meals. If you develop loose stools, divide the dosage so that you take it twice daily, or reduce it slightly.

GABA and L-theanine. Gamma aminobutyric acid is one of the body's main relaxing neurotransmitters and can ease feelings of edginess. Take 500 mg of GABA one to three times daily, at least one hour apart from eating food. Combine it with L-theanine, which boosts the body's production of GABA. Take 200 mg of L-theanine one to three times daily with GABA.

Gamma linolenic acid (GLA). Researchers found that supplements of borage oil, providing 1.3 grams of GLA, help to buffer people against psychological stress. Take 1 to 2 grams daily.

Omega-3 fish oils. The omega-3s, particularly docosahexaenoic acid (DHA), play essential roles in brain development. Although studies have not investigated whether the omega-3 fish oils or DHA would be helpful in PTSD, they are likely to be. Take at least 3 grams daily.

5-HTP. This supplement, 5-hydroxytryptophan, is the immediate precursor to serotonin, the calming neurotransmitter that most psychotropic prescription drugs aim to elevate. Take 50 mg, one to three times daily, apart from meals. If you can purchase L-tryptophan, it has the advantage of being more versatile biochemically. The dosage for L-tryptophan is higher, 500 mg one to three times daily, at least one hour apart from meals.

St. John's wort. This venerable herb (also known as *Hypericum perforatum*) has been used for thousands of years to promote wound healing and treat behavioral disorders. In study after study, St. John's wort has been found to be more effective than the leading antidepressant drugs, including Prozac and Zoloft. In addition, the herb produces fewer side effects than the drugs do. Because depression (the principal use for St. John's wort) is often associated with anxiety in PTSD, the herb may be useful. Take 300 mg of a standardized St. John's wort product three times daily. If you use a tincture, follow the label directions.

Quick Tip

Social Anxiety, Phobia, or Simple Shyness?

In recent years, the medical and the pharmaceutical industries have sought to medicalize many personality quirks. As one example, television commercials promote the drug Paxil (an antidepressant) as a treatment for social anxiety disorder. The drug is supposed to be used to treat people with life-disrupting anxiety about social situations, such as feelings of embarrassment or humiliation.

Sometimes, though, the line between shyness and petrifying anxiety becomes blurred. Certain people are reserved for any number of reasons, and shy people shouldn't be treated as if they have a mental disorder. Nor should a drug prescription be the first line of treatment, when dietary changes or psychological counseling might uncover and correct the source of the problem.

Obsessive-Compulsive Behavior

Each of us has our individual quirks, many of which remain unseen by all but the people who live with us. These habits are usually our most private obsessions and compulsions, and most are innocuous expressions of occasional anxieties. For example, you might keep your coffee table books in neatly aligned piles, repeatedly check to make sure your door is locked, or silently repeat words to yourself until you pronounce them correctly in your own head. Two well-known fictional obsessive-compulsive characters are Detective Adrian Monk from the television show *Monk* and Felix Unger from *The Odd Couple*. Their obsessive-compulsive behavior appears perfectionistic, quirky, ritualistic, and intertwined with details that are lost on other people.

The problems occur when our little obsessions and compulsions start to rule our lives. Sometimes thoughts simply pop into our heads that we have to check, such as, "Did I turn off the headlights?" These obsessive thoughts trigger anxiety, often with a fear that awful consequences will result if we don't check. Compulsive checking or repeating acts reduces that anxiety.

What distinguishes a compulsion is the utter lack of mental or physical pleasure associated with it. Psychologists point out that compulsive behavior is intended to reduce feelings of anxiety, not to make us feel good. Usually, a person who is obsessive-compulsive is driven to perform the anxiety-reducing compulsion. Here are some examples of common obsessive-compulsive acts:

Checking. This may be the most prevalent form of obsessive-compulsive behavior. Common activities include repeatedly checking that a door is locked, that the stove has been turned off, or that a letter hasn't gotten stuck in a mailbox. This behavior can also include checking e-mail late at night or while on vacation. In serious types of obsessive-compulsive behavior, people might perform checks dozens of times each day.

Fear of contamination. Some people may clean doorknobs, drinking glasses, and computer keyboards that other people have touched. One of the most common contamination-related anxieties is repeated hand washing that, in severe cases, results in raw and bleeding skin.

Repeated acts. Touching an object over and over again, such as a button on your car CD player, or touching a certain number of times (to ensure either an even or an odd number of touches) is another type of obsessive-compulsive behavior. Under some circumstances, repeatedly thanking God (in your head, nonverbally) also reflects obsessive-compulsiveness.

Hoarding or collecting. More than simply being pack rats, some people find it impossible to throw anything away. Obsessive-compulsive hoarders may have homes or apartments that look like junk shops or storage sheds. An extreme example is a person who, over many years, has kept thousands of newspapers and magazines—so many that paths between rooms are practically like tunnels. More minor examples of obsessive-compulsive acts include needless hoarding, such as keeping hundreds of rubber bands in a kitchen drawer (rationalized, for example, by saying you'll donate them to a charitable organization, as if it really needs those rubber bands).

Frugality. There's nothing wrong with being careful how you spend your money, but obsessive-compulsive people can take frugality to an extreme. For example, washing plastic food bags for reuse until they tatter is a form of obsessive-compulsive behavior.

Psychological Tips

Obsessive-compulsive behavior can be reduced through cognitive behavioral therapy, which coaches patients how to ignore, stop, or control their obsessive and compulsive impulses. The objective of these therapies is to set up psychological trip wires so that people immediately recognize and challenge their obsessive-compulsive acts.

If your obsessive-compulsive habit is checking, make a list of things you routinely check, such as the door, stove, lamp, or headlights. Apply what you've already learned about being mindful, and resolve to pay special attention when you lock the door or turn off the stove, lamp, or headlights. Later, when you develop an obsession about the object, remind yourself that you already make a point of checking it and that you don't need to check again.

Recognize that your obsessive-compulsive habits are irrational impulses and that you don't have to respond to them. Initially, this approach may increase your anxiety, but you may lessen it by giving yourself a distraction, such as a magazine, crossword puzzle, or television show. You'll realize that nothing bad will happen to you by not checking or repeating.

Find a healthy outlet for your obsessive-compulsive tendencies. Many creative pursuits and hobbies benefit from an attention to detail that is practically obsessive-compulsive in nature. Such activities may siphon off or focus some of the anxiety that predisposes you toward irrational obsessive-compulsive habits. You can become a meticulous collector—so long, of course, as that hoarding doesn't become another obsessive-compulsive habit.

Eating Habits

Maintaining stable blood sugar levels and reducing overall anxiety levels will help to lessen obsessive-compulsive behavior. Therefore, follow my eating plan in chapter 5. Emphasize protein-rich foods and high-fiber vegetables, while avoiding fast foods and sugary foods. It's especially important to give up coffee and alcohol.

Helpful Supplements

B-complex vitamins. Researchers recently reported that obsessive-compulsive behavior was strongly associated with high blood levels of homocysteine, a marker of low folic acid intake. Vitamins B3 and B12 may also help to treat obsessive-compulsive disorder. Because B vitamins are largely synergistic, I typically recommend the entire B-complex. Start with a high-potency B-complex (or a high-potency multivitamin) supplement containing 25 to 50 mg of vitamins B1, B2, and B3. To this, consider adding 500 mg of vitamin B3 (niacinamide), 1,000 mcg of folic acid, and 500 mcg of sublingual (under the tongue) vitamin B12. *Note*: Again, take B vitamins in the morning or the early afternoon, with food, not in the evening.

Dimethylglycine (DMG). This nutrientlike substance is a precursor to glycine, an amino acid and a calming neurotransmitter. Some evidence suggests that DMG might help to reduce compulsive behavior. It has also been used to treat behavioral problems in autistic children. Take 125 mg two to three times daily. If DMG causes hyperactive behavior, adding 800 mg of folic acid (a B vitamin) with each DMG supplement may lessen this side effect.

Glycine. This amino acid (protein building block) has the simplest chemical structure of any amino acid—and it may have some of the most diverse roles. It is a relaxing neurotransmitter that has anti-inflammatory and cell-protective properties. It also blunts the postmeal increase in blood sugar levels, thereby lowering the risk of diabetes.

N-acetylcysteine. This amino acid antioxidant and compound appears to safely modify the activity of glutamate, a neurotransmitter. In reports of obsessive compulsiveness and self-mutilation, Yale University physicians reported that NAC led to significant improvements. The dosage used was 600 mg twice daily.

Inositol. Several studies have found that supplemental inositol helps to reduce obsessive-compulsive behavior. In a six-week clinical trial, 18 grams daily cut both obsessive and compulsive behavior by about half. As I noted in the previous section, this dosage can probably be decreased to 6 to 8 grams daily by combining inositol with B-complex vitamins.

5-HTP. Because serotonin-regulating antidepressant drugs often provide some benefits in obsessive-compulsive behavior, 5-HTP or L-tryptophan is also likely to help. It may take as long as six months for these nutrients to have a noticeable effect. If you use 5-HTP, take 50 mg one to three times daily, apart from meals. If you use L-tryptophan, take 500 mg one to three times daily, at least one hour apart from meals.

Sage. This culinary herb has potent mood-enhancing properties. Although common sage (*Salvia officinalis*) is the most widely used, Spanish sage (*Salvia lavandulaefolia*) has a stronger flavor and is probably safer in high dosages. In a recent study, British researchers found that supplemental Spanish sage had "striking" effects on mood. The herb helped subjects to feel more alert, calm, and contented, which might have moderated obsessive-compulsive tendencies.

In the next chapter, I'll focus on impulsive and distractible behavior, which possesses some elements of anxiety, panic, and obsessive-compulsiveness.

10

Reducing Distractible and Impulsive ADHD-like Behavior

Many people in modern society seem distracted, impulsive, bored, or addicted to certain types of distractible behavior. These traits are often ascribed to children with attention-deficit-hyperactivity disorder (ADHD). Today, many children with ADHD have become adults with either ADHD or ADHD-like symptoms because they do not consume adequate neuronutrients. The problem with this type of behavior is that it reduces our ability to clearly focus, hurts our productivity and relationships, and, at times, it risks serious injury.

This ADHD-like behavior has also been described as "continuous partial attention" by Linda Stone, a former executive at Apple and Microsoft. When she spoke at the Emerging Technology Conference in San Diego early in 2006, she (like the other speakers) was competing with the audience's use of e-mail, Web surfing, and text messaging. It was an eerie reflection of much of our society. Increasingly, people devote just a little attention to each of their multitasking activities, not giving full attention to any of them.

I'll describe several examples of this odd behavior. One is the person who is either engaged in a face-to-face conversation or is sitting or walking by himself. He pulls out his cell phone and begins scrolling through its features, not because it's ringing but because he's bored or anxious. He is not in the moment or paying attention to his surroundings.

As another example, consider drivers who occupy themselves with any number of distractions—talking on a cell phone, eating, or applying makeup. If you ask them why they do all of these things, they may say that they don't otherwise have enough time, that they feel as though they're being efficient, or that driving is boring—as if driving a couple thousand pounds of metal at high speed weren't important enough to focus on. Or they may simply stare at you as if *you* are the one with a problem. Such people are also addicted to their distractions.

In October and November 2005, a bank robber in the suburbs of Washington, D.C., took distractibility to new heights. In each of four robberies, the young woman gave tellers a note demanding money, then walked out of the bank—all while continuing to talk on her cell phone! She may have been too distracted by her cell phone to be mindful of the array of security cameras at the banks. A photograph of her chatting on a cell phone during a holdup was published in newspapers around the country, and soon after that, she was arrested.

One of the most common ways that distractibility and impulsiveness play out in modern society is with our eating habits. With plenty to do at home and at work, people often don't plan ahead for substantial, healthy meals. So when we do get hungry (that is, when our blood sugar is low and we're already short on neuronutrients), we are especially susceptible to making impulsive decisions about where to quickly get our next meal—such as choosing between the drive-through line at McDonald's or at Taco Bell. In a real sense, eating has become an impulsive act. Unfortunately, meals and soft drinks that are high in refined carbohydrates, sugars, and unhealthful fats make the situation worse.

Distractible, Impulsive, and Addictive Behavior

Changes in our work and social habits, as well as in our eating habits, have contributed to the prevalence of distractible and impulsive behavior in adults. These behavior patterns have been sometimes described as adult ADHD. Some characteristics of this cluster of distractible-impulsive-addiction behavior include

- Feeling restless or hyper—having difficulty sitting still for long periods
- Being impulsive—acting on sudden urges or desires
- Being addicted to impulsive acts—frequently feeling the need to impulsively check or to seek distractions
- Being easily distracted—using a variety of activities (such as checking e-mail) to interrupt primary work or tasks
- Having poor concentration and memory—having difficulty focusing on a single task for a long time

In this chapter, I describe some of the nutrisocial factors that shape these behaviors, and I suggest ways to reduce them. As you might expect, diet and supplements can often completely reverse the behaviors.

Impulsive Behavior

Impulse shopping is one of the most common forms of impulsive behavior. Large retailers use various techniques—from displays and lighting to background music—to tempt shoppers into making purchases. When we see products at a store that really appeal to us, perhaps an article of clothing or a sleek new electronic gadget, we may fantasize about owning it and imagine how cool it would make us look. With a swipe of a credit card, it belongs to us.

Over the last twenty years, impulsive and excessive shopping has increased, as evidenced by the huge amount of high-interest consumer credit-card debt in the United States. We are more likely to make hasty and expensive decisions because we don't give them enough thought.

Multitasking has helped to foster impulsive behavior. Doing more than one thing at a time has become so instilled that, when we are limited to doing just one thing, we often don't feel right. Around 100 B.C., the Roman philosopher Publilius Syrus observed, "To do two things at once is to do neither." Multitasking is not a new phenomenon. It has just gotten a lot worse.

Researchers have found that intense multitasking triggers a classic stress response, including an elevation of adrenaline and cortisol levels.

So, instead of reducing stress, multitasking actually increases stress. Furthermore, sustained high levels of stress hormones damage brain cells that are involved in forming new memories. So if you seem more spacey when stressed, it's because you are losing some of your ability to concentrate and remember. The simple fact is that we cannot focus equally on each task when we multitask; we are distracted by the other tasks we are doing.

Impulsiveness is a classic symptom of ADHD in children. Instead of darting in front of cars, however, impulsive adults spend their days darting about mentally or physically. They have difficulty thinking before acting, and they accomplish far less than they might otherwise. Their impulsive behavior can even lead to dangerous acts, such as running red lights.

Distractibility and Poor Focus

Just as multitasking encourages our minds to flit between activities, it also promotes attention overload, distractibility, and poor focus. In analyzing multitasking at a financial-services business, Gloria Mark, Ph.D., of the University of California, Irvine, found that the typical employee jumps from one task to another every three minutes and gets interrupted every two minutes. Multitasking promotes distractibility and hyper behavior, and in the process, we lose the ability to filter out less important stimuli to keep us on track.

Through all this, our attention spans seem to become shorter and shorter—another characteristic of ADHD. In 1998, we delighted in surfing the Internet, even with slow download speeds. Then, after we got a taste of how fast download speeds could be at work, we felt that we had to have equally fast download times at home. As a result, we've become impatient with dial-up modems. People now expect to surf Internet sites as fast as they switch channels on television—but not everything in the world happens at a snap of the fingers.

Like multitasking, cell phones have significantly increased our distractibility (and, of course, we often multitask with cell phones). When cell phones first became widely popular in the 1990s, many people reacted with bumper stickers that said "Hang Up and Drive." Today, we might benefit from signs saying "Hang Up and Walk," as people wander distracted through supermarkets, pace the sidewalks in front of bookstores, and cross streets oblivious to everything around them.

Impulsive-Addictive Behavior

The blend of impulsiveness and distractibility has set the stage for what could best be described as impulsive-addictive behavior. Similar to being addicted to alcohol or drugs, getting a hit triggers the release of neurochemicals, including endorphins, adrenaline, or dopamine. Withdrawal, the phase when levels of these neurochemicals decline, results in a feeling of uneasiness or outright anxiety. Because of these uncomfortable post-hit feelings, we can become addicted to activities that prompt a quick surge of these neurochemicals.

Gambling is perhaps the oldest and best-known form of impulsive-addictive behavior. Las Vegas casinos have perfected the art of addictive environments with dizzying arrays of flashing lights and the ka-ching sound of silver dollars to attract and maintain the attention of gamblers. The sights and sounds of casinos would be the perfect sensory environment to stimulate ADHD in children. For adults, the setting is well orchestrated to overstimulate the senses and encourage other addictive behaviors, such as smoking and drinking alcohol.

Certain symptoms of Internet addiction are similar to those in other types of addictive behavior. These include cravings (in this case, for more time on the computer), neglecting family members and friends, moodiness when not using the computer, and lying to people about the amount of time spent on the Internet. In a newspaper story, a twenty-two-year-old man described why he kept his e-mail and instant-messaging connection active twenty-four hours a day: "I may not use it, but it could ring anytime. . . . If I don't have it, I feel cut off."

One danger with Internet addiction, like any type of addiction, is that it can interfere with normal and healthy interactions between people. It literally becomes a distraction from the rest of one's life, and the implications go beyond the occasional Internet affair that leads to a divorce. When we spend excessive time on the computer and not interacting with another person face to face, we find it all too easy to forget how to engage in stimulating conversations, use good manners while eating, or show common courtesies to other people. Our focus shifts to maintaining obsessive-compulsive or impulsive-addictive behavior.

The problem is not just Internet addiction or even paying more attention to a cell phone conversation than to driving or walking. New personal technologies often breed serious distractions by encouraging implusive-addictive behaviors. The user attempts to multitask but inevitably focuses more on interacting with the technology than with real human beings. In November 2005, a teenager in suburban Denver was text messaging on his cell phone while driving his car—and swerved into the bicycle lane and killed a cyclist. This goes beyond immaturity, a lack of focus, or stupidity. It's a brain incapable of sound judgment because of unbalanced neuronutrients and neurotransmitters.

Research on addictive behaviors has zeroed in specifically on the neurotransmitter dopamine (described in chapter 3), which plays important roles in pleasure, motivation, thinking, and physical activity. Eating tasty food and having sex elevate dopamine levels. So does the thrill of shopping, sometimes referred to as a "shopper's high."

In terms of neurochemistry, addictive behaviors are similar to addictive drugs. For example, cocaine works in large part by boosting dopamine levels in the brain. The drug blocks the normal breakdown of dopamine, thereby maintaining higher levels of the neurotransmitter. The sense of euphoria induced by these drugs is actually related to high dopamine levels, but it's the cocaine that artificially creates those high levels. Underlying the addiction to cocaine is an addiction to dopamine.

Sometimes L-dopa, a dopamine-boosting drug used to treat Parkinson's disease, can lead to bizarre behavior. According to a report in the *Archives of Neurology*, a dopamine-enhancing drug (pramipexole) sometimes leads to compulsive gambling. In one case, a patient treated with the drug started playing the slot machines at a casino near his home, losing thousands of dollars a day for two years. As soon as the drug was stopped or its dosage reduced, the compulsive gambling stopped.

The addictive nature of dopamine seems to require glutamate, a dietary amino acid that can be neurotoxic in large amounts. In addition, some people inherit genetic variations that may predispose them to addictions. For example, one variation in the gene that programs a cellular dopamine receptor (which the neurotransmitter attaches to on brain cells) is associated with an especially strong addiction to nicotine and more difficulty breaking a tobacco habit.

Psychological Tips

The benefits of supplements and dietary improvements in reducing distractible and impulsive behavior are so impressive that relatively few behavioral tips may be needed. Often, supplements lead to a clearheaded, focused, and calm feeling. Still, here are several tips.

Learn to disengage. Develop an inner switch that alerts you when you see yourself start to act impulsively or in an impulsive-addictive manner. For example, if you're shopping, out to dinner, or socializing with friends, you don't have to answer your cell phone. If you feel restless, which can be a prelude to impulsive actions, look for one calming activity, such as reading a book or a magazine or listening to music. The more you use this inner switch, the better you will become at resisting impulses.

Resist the impulse. When you find yourself beginning to slip into impulsive-addictive behavior, consciously resist the pattern. This may generate a little anxiety at first, but you will likely get better at it so that you mentally note but otherwise ignore the impulse.

Be mindful. To focus and improve your memory, you have to first pay attention. In today's world, this often means consciously ignoring potential distractions, such as trying to do too many things at once. Stick to doing what you have to do until you finish it. If it's a time-consuming project, you can give yourself a break after an hour or two and work on something else. That kind of work shifting may actually sharpen your concentration.

Eating Habits

Follow my dietary guidelines in chapter 5, but place greater emphasis on eating fresh fish, which are high in omega-3 fats. Modern processed foods—what you buy at fast-food restaurants or in packages for use at home—are generally rich in highly refined omega-6 fats and contain virtually no omega-3 fats. Historically, the ratio between these families of fats was approximately 1:1. With food processing, the omega-6 fats overwhelm the omega-3 fats by a ratio of about 30:1.

To correct this situation, you must do more than simply increase your intake of fish or take omega-3 fish oils. You must eliminate virtually all foods containing processed omega-6s, including most cooking oils (such as corn, safflower, peanut, and soybean oils), salad dressings, microwave meals, and deep-fried foods (such as French fries, fried chicken, and fried fish). By dutifully following these guidelines and taking the fish and plant oil supplements recommended in the following pages, your body's fatty acid ratios should normalize after several months.

For cooking oils, stick with olive oil and macadamia nut oil. Because omega-6 fats are essential, you can obtain what you need by eating raw nuts and seeds, such as almonds and sunflower seeds.

Helpful Supplements

Dietary fatty acids. Many different essential dietary fats have a profound effect on impulsive, distractible, and aggressive behavior. These fats include the omega-3 fish oils, specifically eicosapentaenoic acid (EPA) and docosahexaenoic acid (DHA), as well as the omega-6 plant oil gamma linolenic acid (GLA). These fats are best known for their anti-inflammatory effects, but they also play a major role in brain development and the brain's responses to stress.

A recent study found that the by-products of these fats control stress-induced impulsive behavior. In a study of children with behavioral disorders, researchers found that a combination of omega-3 fish oils and GLA (in a 4:1 ratio) led to significant reductions in impulsive and hyperactive behavior and better focus, reflected in improved reading and spelling. Considerable other research has confirmed that EPA, DHA, and GLA help a wide range of impulsive behaviors. One researcher has suggested that DHA, because of its integral role in nerve tissue, can normalize "excitability" across the board.

For impulsive and distractible behavior in adults, start by taking 3 grams of omega-3 fish oils and 200 to 500 mg of GLA. (The GLA will be derived from borage, evening primrose, or black currant seed oils—the dosage is more important than the source.) You may increase the dosages to 6 grams of omega-3 fish oils and 1,000 mg (1 gram) of GLA. Follow the other supplement recommendations in the order described.

GABA. Gamma aminobutyric acid, both an amino acid and a neurotransmitter, helps the brain to filter out nonessential information—that is, distractions. Impulsive behavior often entails responding to nonessential and distracting stimuli, and it is likely that GABA will be of benefit. Take 500 mg one to three times daily.

Pycnogenol. This antioxidant complex, extracted from the bark of French maritime pine trees, contains around forty compounds. Some reports, published and anecdotal, have found it helpful in treating distractibility, impulsiveness, and hyperactivity in children. It may have similar benefits in adults. Try 100 mg twice daily.

B-complex vitamins. By now, you understand how important a foundation B vitamins are for healthy neurotransmitter levels and activity. Take a high-potency B-complex (or a high-potency multivitamin) containing 25 to 50 mg of vitamins B1, B2, and B3. If your diet has tended to be high in sugars and carbohydrates, add 100 mg of additional vitamin B1. *Note*: Take B vitamins in the morning or the early afternoon, with food.

Magnesium and vitamin B6. In a French study, researchers found that a combination of supplemental magnesium and vitamin B6 reduces poor attention, twitchiness, physical aggression, and moodiness in children. Adults would likely benefit as well. For adults, take 400 to 600 mg of magnesium citrate daily (divided into two doses with meals) and 100 mg of vitamin B6. You can take this amount of vitamin B6 in addition to a high-potency B-complex supplement.

DHEA. The hormone dehydroepiandrosterone is the precursor to estrogen and testosterone. Some evidence suggests that supplemental DHEA may reduce cocaine addiction, and it may have similar benefits in lessening addictive behavior that does not involve drugs or alcohol. Although DHEA is available at many health food stores without a prescription, it's best to have your doctor measure your blood DHEA-S levels to ensure that you need the hormone. If your levels are low to low normal, consider adding 25 mg of DHEA daily. Have your doctor check your blood levels again after six months. *Note*: If you are under thirty-five years of age, it's unlikely that you need DHEA supplementation.

Ginseng. Extracts of ginseng (specifically, those containing saponins) appear to modulate dopamine levels in the brain. In a study of nicotine addiction, researchers found that ginseng extracts decreased the nicotine-induced activation of dopamine. The same mechanism may apply to nondrug-related addictive behavior. Ginseng is certainly worth trying for thirty days. Follow the label directions for use because potencies vary among manufacturers.

N-acetylcysteine. NAC may help to restore normal brain levels of glutamate, a calming neurotransmitter that is also needed for GABA production. A study found that high doses of NAC (600 mg four times daily) diminished interest in and desire for cocaine. Along with some of the other supplements recommended, consider adding 500 to 1,000 mg daily. *Note*: Because of its high sulfur content, NAC has a rotten-egg odor. Take the supplement without sniffing it.

11

The Overweight-Prediabetes Connection to Mood Swings

You've probably noticed that your mood can quickly turn sour when you're hungry or tired. At these times, you're more likely to be impatient, irritable, cranky, and prone to anger. You might even feel a little dizzy or physically shaky. If you drive to and from work, consider how you feel during the late afternoon commute home, when you're tired and hungry and don't have much patience for being a courteous driver. The truth is that being overweight or prediabetic makes you even more hungry and can affect your moods.

What's happening inside your body? Both hunger and tiredness are often signs of low blood sugar (glucose), fairly quick or extreme shifts between high and low glucose levels, or other difficulties dealing with carbohydrates and sugars. In some people, changes in blood sugar can lead to sudden and dramatic mood swings or overreactions, such as feeling sick and tired of something or losing your cool. Blood sugar problems can also lead to being mentally fuzzy or spacey.

The body and the brain function best when blood sugar levels are within a fairly narrow and relatively stable range. When we regularly consume sugars and sugarlike carbohydrates, however, our ability to deal with these foods breaks down. This deterioration occurs faster in some people than in others, but it is now common because foods based on refined sugars and carbohydrates have become the dietary mainstay of many Americans.

Historically, people ate few if any of these pure sugars and carbohydrates. Biologically, we're not designed to handle them. Today, though, the average American consumes about 150 pounds of refined sugars each year, along with 400 pounds or so of refined carbohydrates. These refined carbohydrates have been heavily processed and are absorbed rapidly, very much like sugars.

Most people are unaware of the huge amount of sugars they consume. That's because sugars are added to foods and beverages before they reach the grocery store (or restaurant, as the case may be). For example, a 12-ounce soft drink contains approximately ten teaspoons of sugars (usually, sucrose or high-fructose corn syrup), and a 64-ounce soft drink averages one-half pound of sugars.

The physical and mental consequences of eating all of these sugars and sugarlike carbohydrates may sometimes take years to develop, and they contribute to a variety of intertwined health problems, including obesity, diabetes, and heart disease. Although sugary foods are often promoted as energy foods, whatever increase in energy they provide is short-lived, followed by a speedy drop in energy levels and often mood.

Mood Swings, Tiredness, Mental Fuzziness, and Overweight

People with mood swings are frequently described as having unpredictable, changeable, mercurial, or Jekyll-and-Hyde personalities. They may be pleasant one moment and irritable, mean, or depressed the next. Sometimes, a moody person will overreact with anger to another person's innocent comment. Tiredness and mental fuzziness are often part of the picture. Tiredness is a persistent feeling of fatigue, although the person does almost everything that is expected at work and home. Mental fuzziness is characterized by difficulty in concentrating and remembering. Although tiredness might seem to set the stage for mood changes, blood sugar problems are the source of both problems.

What You Should Know

Mood swings, chronic feelings of tiredness, and mental fuzziness are commonly signs of underlying (and often undiagnosed) blood sugar disorders, including impaired glucose tolerance, insulin resistance, metabolic syndrome, Syndrome X, prediabetes, and full-blown diabetes. Along the spectrum of glucose intolerance—perhaps more accurately described as sugar and carbohydrate intolerance—people may display a range of mood and behavior problems.

A number of clues point to underlying sugar and carbohydrate intolerance. Among them are

- Regular consumption of fast foods, convenience foods, and soft drinks
- Eating habits that include a lot of sweet snacks
- Cravings for sugary or carbohydrate-rich foods, such as sweets
- Feeling good after eating sugary or carbohydrate-rich foods
- Feeling lousy when you can't eat sugary or carbohydrate-rich foods
- Overeating or eating large portion sizes
- Excessive intake of alcoholic beverages, especially beer and spirits
- Routinely feeling tired and having difficulty getting out of bed
- Being overweight, especially if much of the weight is around the belly
- Rapidly changeable moods

Blood sugar problems may not always be the sole cause of mood swings. When they are not the apparent cause, they are usually an aggravating factor. The moods of some individuals can literally fluctuate with the ups and downs of their blood sugar levels. When glucose levels are low, the activity of higher brain areas decreases, allowing more primitive and aggressive behavior to be expressed. (In some people, however, blood sugar disorders may not affect mood at all.) Alcohol can exacerbate the problem by reducing inhibitions and encouraging us to ignore social constraints, which is why drunks often become physically aggressive.

Mood swings, tiredness, and mental fuzziness are often intertwined with being overweight, and excess body fat is one sign of problematic eating habits and blood sugar levels. If you are overweight, even by as little as ten pounds, you are more likely than a thin person to have blood sugar problems, and you also have an extremely high risk of developing full-blown diabetes within five to ten years. The scale of this problem in the United States is enormous, and it's growing in Western Europe and other developed and developing nations. One-third of Americans are overweight, and another third are obese—that is, weighing thirty pounds or more than their ideal weight. Yet being thin doesn't make you immune to blood sugar problems. As I noted in my best-selling book *Syndrome X: The Complete Nutritional Program to Prevent and Reverse Insulin Resistance*, 25 percent of thin people have signs of prediabetes.

The excessive consumption of refined sugars and carbohydrates has set the stage for this tangle of mood, behavioral, and physical problems. Here's why. Under normal circumstances—that is, when we eat protein and high-fiber nonstarchy vegetables—our blood sugar increases moderately and the body responds by secreting the hormone insulin. This hormone helps to transport blood sugar into cells, where it should be burned for energy.

When we consume large quantities of refined sugars and carbohydrates, the result is an exaggerated and abnormal response. Refined sugars and carbohydrates are rapidly digested, prompting a sharp increase in blood sugar levels. Because very high blood sugar levels are toxic to the kidneys, the body responds by secreting large amounts of insulin to rein in the blood sugar. Insulin helps to convert excess blood sugar to fat, particularly belly fat. In addition, some people secrete especially large amounts of insulin, which may cause a precipitous drop in their blood sugar levels—and mood.

After people eat refined sugars and carbohydrates for a number of years, their cells start to ignore, or resist, insulin's effects, leading to a condition known as insulin resistance—the hallmark of prediabetes and diabetes. Recent research strongly suggests that insulin resistance can develop in brain cells. Although this research has focused on how cerebral insulin resistance promotes overeating, obesity, and diabetes, it is likely that it would also affect mood and behavior.

The time line for developing insulin resistance varies from person to person, but its prevalence has increased substantially in younger adults and now children, leading to the earlier development of obesity and diabetes. As people become more resistant to insulin, their blood sugar levels remain elevated and they will be more likely to develop fat around the belly. In fact, insulin is widely considered the "fat-storage" hormone. When blood sugar levels are elevated, a person is more likely to have difficulty concentrating and to become fuzzy minded—all well-known signs of diabetes. Insulin has many other undesirable effects, such as increasing blood pressure, cholesterol, and triglyceride levels, all of which I describe in my *Syndrome X* book.

The situation grows worse with time. As glucose tolerance decreases, so does our ability to taste sweetness in food. In response, we tend to add more sugar to our coffee, crave sweets, or eat increasingly rich desserts. As our blood sugar and insulin levels become more abnormal, we're also more likely to feel tired—and more tempted to eat sugary foods or to drink caffeinated beverages to increase our energy levels. Of course, the more sugar and refined carbohydrates we eat, the more problematic our blood sugar and insulin levels become.

Eating Habits

Correcting problems with blood sugar will often reduce moodiness and sharpen thinking. Weight loss usually follows as an additional benefit, because hunger jags and cravings usually diminish, leading to less eating.

The primary approach to correcting blood sugar disorders is dietary. First, rule out food allergies. The most likely allergies involve wheat- and dairy-containing foods, although corn and soy may also be problematic.

Follow my dietary advice in chapter 5. Emphasize healthful sources of protein, such as fish, chicken, and turkey, along with high-fiber and nonstarchy vegetables. These foods tend to stabilize blood sugar and insulin levels. You'll have to eat fresh foods or minimally processed frozen foods (such as cooking frozen chicken breasts or steaming frozen vegetables).

Avoid eating microwave meals, most other packaged foods, and anything from fast-food restaurants. If you are overweight or discover that you are especially sensitive to sugars and carbohydrates, you may have to eliminate nearly all starchy and carb-containing foods. You might be able to eat small amounts of brown rice, however, if the rice is buffered by protein and high-fiber vegetables.

Although it sounds more like folklore than science, vinegar can reduce appetite and improve both blood sugar and insulin levels. Several recent studies by reputable researchers have shown this to be the case. The acetic acid in vinegar inhibits the activity of various carbohydrate-digesting enzymes, including amylase, sucrase, maltase, and lactase. Basically, vinegar is a natural starch and sugar blocker. When these enzymes are blocked, sugars and starches pass through the digestive tract in much the way that indigestible fiber does. You can use vinegar in a quick homemade salad dressing. See chapter 5 for the recipe.

Psychological Tips

Mood swings related to fluctuating blood sugar levels are largely biological, not psychological, in nature. It helps to be tuned in to the early signs of hunger, fatigue, and deteriorating moods, however, so that you can sidestep a crash in your moods or behavior. Get in the habit of keeping some protein (such as deli turkey) or complex carbohydrates (such as your own trail nut mix) handy. Snack on these foods when you sense your blood sugar levels dropping and your mood starting to change.

The up-and-down nature of these mood swings often resembles an addiction cycle. If you have become dependent on eating junk foods, you have to wean yourself from those habits. It's often easier doing that cold turkey instead of slowly. When you eliminate all of the problematic foods, you may have several uncomfortable days with feelings of hunger, headaches, and possibly other symptoms. Most people start to clear by the beginning of the fifth day and then feel better than they have in years. In some ways, you may have to view junk foods the way Alcoholics Anonymous views alcohol: one bite is too many, and a thousand is not enough.

Nearly everyone goes off his or her diet or strays from healthy eating habits on occasion. This is not a moral failure. Sugary foods are tasty and tempting; however, it's important that you resume more healthful eating habits as quickly as possible. Because of the addictive nature of sugary foods, you may again have to break a food addiction.

Helpful Supplements

Several nutritional supplements can enhance insulin function, promote chemical reactions that burn (rather than store) glucose, and dampen appetite. Yet these supplements will probably not by themselves lead to any substantial loss of weight. You need to make dietary changes to achieve significant weight loss. Take these supplements with your meals.

alphabetic. If you are diabetic or prediabetic and averse to taking a lot of pills, including nutritional supplements, consider taking alphabetic. This once-a-day vitamin/mineral supplement was formulated for people with prediabetes and diabetes. The overall dosage of ingredients is modest, so it is unlikely to interact with any diabetic medications. (See ordering information in the appendix.)

Alpha-lipoic acid. This vitaminlike nutrient has been used for decades in Germany to treat the complications of diabetes. It improves the efficiency of insulin, allowing less of the hormone to do its job. (With respect to insulin, less is usually better.) Some studies have also found that it can lower blood sugar levels. These mechanisms would lead to more stable blood sugar levels and decreased appetite.

Researchers recently discovered that alpha-lipoic acid plays a key role in regulating hunger and therefore appetite and weight. When cell levels of glucose or fat decrease, activity of the enzyme AMP-activated protein kinase (AMPK) increases. AMPK governs sugar and fat metabolism. In experiments with laboratory rats, researchers found that supplemental alpha-lipoic acid reduced AMPK activity, which led to less food intake, lower body weight, and lower blood levels of glucose and insulin.

The therapeutic dosage for treating diabetic neuropathy, a nerve disease, is 200 mg of alpha-lipoic acid three times daily. In glucose intolerance and other forms of prediabetes, 100 to 300 mg daily should be helpful. You can combine it with the supplements discussed further on.

Insulow. This product provides R-lipoic acid (the more biologically active form of the antioxidant) combined with the B vitamin biotin. Both nutrients enhance insulin function and glucose utilization. The product may be of particular benefit to people with prediabetes and diabetes. Follow the label directions for use. (See ordering information in the appendix.)

Chromium. This essential mineral is needed for the normal functioning of insulin, and studies have found that it can lower blood sugar levels. Take 400 to 1,000 mcg of chromium picolinate daily by itself, and about 400 to 500 mg daily if you combine it with other supplements described here.

Cinnamon. Consuming small amounts of cinnamon, in foods or supplements, can greatly improve blood sugar levels. In one study, researchers gave cinnamon to 60 overweight people with type 2 diabetes. The dosages were 1, 3, or 6 grams daily for 40 days. People taking cinnamon had decreases in blood sugar ranging from 18 to 29 percent. Although you can buy cinnamon in capsules, it is far less expensive to purchase the ground spice and sprinkle it on oatmeal or fruit, such as apples, cantaloupe, or berries. Take 1 to 6 grams daily. One gram of cinnamon is about one-quarter teaspoon of the spice, so 4 grams would equal 1 teaspoonful.

Ginseng. Several studies have found that American ginseng (*Panax quinquefolius*) can lower glucose levels in both diabetics and nondiabetic subjects by 20 to 38 percent. Dosages in these studies have ranged from 1 to 3 grams daily, with higher dosages having a greater benefit.

Silymarin. People with serious blood sugar problems may benefit greatly from silymarin, an antioxidant extract of the herb milk thistle (*Silybum marianum*). Silymarin is widely used to enhance function of the liver, which works in tandem with the pancreas to regulate glucose levels. In a twelve-month study of seriously ill diabetic patients, 600 mg daily of silymarin reduced glucose in diabetics by 9.5 to 15 percent. The patients also benefited from lower levels of sugar in the urine, glycated hemoglobin, and insulin requirements.

12

Dealing with Down Days, Depression, and Bipolar Disorder

epression is the most widely recognized mood disorder, thanks to the widespread advertising of antidepressant medications. Unfortunately, these medications don't correct the underlying biochemical or psychological causes of depression, and they often pose serious side effects.

What exactly is depression? The simplest definition is sadness plus hopelessness—that is, a deep sense of sadness combined with a feeling that life won't get better. Serious bouts of depression affect approximately one in every five people at least once in their lives, and having one episode of serious depression greatly increases the chances of experiencing subsequent episodes.

Rather than being a single disorder, depression occurs in various intensities. Adding to the complexity, depression can have multiple intertwined causes. For example, some cases of depression are triggered by grief resulting from the death of a family member or a friend, from divorce, or from losing a job. Grief is a powerful stressor, and it can significantly alter neurotransmitter levels and activity. If people don't make a concerted effort to rejuvenate their health and their neurotransmitters, these changes in brain chemistry may be very slow to normalize. In addition, some people inherit a genetic susceptibility to serious, long-term depression. For other people, feelings of depression seem to descend like a cloud without any apparent triggering event. In these cases, the depression is probably due strictly to nutritional or biochemical imbalances.

Depression is commonly associated with a diagnosis of serious diseases, such as diabetes, heart disease, and cancer. Doctors refer to this as "comorbid depression" because it coexists with morbidity (a medical term for disease). Again, the grief or shock of hearing a serious diagnosis may trigger profound changes in neurotransmitter levels. Yet disease-associated depression is not only caused by a serious medical diagnosis. Chronic feelings of depression actually increase the risk of *developing* these diseases—perhaps because they share some common nutritional and biochemical underpinnings.

Considerable research has shown that depression can result from a low intake of B-complex vitamins, such as folic acid and vitamins B6

How Peter Dealt with His Depression

Peter was an exceptionally creative person who was a bad fit for his job as a technical writer and editor. He was unhappy with his job, but because of the demands of his new family, he had little time to look for other work. Then, one day he hit bottom. As he was editing a poorly written document, he felt a sudden and overwhelming sense of depression, as if he were slowly drowning.

After telephoning his wife and describing how he felt, Peter resolved to start looking for a new job or other work options. After several months of research and talking with magazine editors and potential corporate clients, Peter realized that he could make at least as much money as a full-time freelance writer.

Although the transition to self-employment was scary, Peter quickly discovered that it was the right decision. In the first year of working for himself, he made more money than he ever did working in a corporate setting. He was also able to work at home and had more time for himself and his family. He hasn't felt depressed since.

and B12. It is related to high levels of homocysteine, a risk factor for heart disease that is connected with low B-vitamin levels. Indeed, Glucophage (metformin) and Prilosec (omeprazole) interfere with the body's use of B vitamins and other nutrients. Another dietary clue is that being overweight and insulin resistant (prediabetic) increases the odds of experiencing depression.

Waking Up to Down Days

Down or blue days describe occasional feelings of depression without any obvious triggering life event. You might feel a bit subdued, unmotivated about work, or as if you've got the "blahs." Usually, the down mood lifts after a day or two.

What You Should Know

It's normal to occasionally experience a down or blue day. Sometimes it feels a little like your body and your mind are tapping gently on the brakes, especially if you have been working hard for several weeks or months.

As an example, I experience a down day once or twice a year. Instead of trying to push against it or work at my usual deadline-oriented pace, I've learned to use these days to do more routine tasks, such as cleaning my office or filing papers. I have also found that the occasional down day is a wonderful time for contemplation, allowing me to reflect about what I like and what I want to change in my life. My down days don't seem to occur with any rhyme or reason, other than the fact that they usually appear after I've been working very hard for several straight months.

If your down feelings last for two weeks or more, or if you seem to have down days regularly, you may have a more serious form of depression. If that's the case, read the rest of this chapter and consider whether any specific frustrations or life events might have led up to these feelings. Above all, make an appointment with a nutritionally oriented physician or psychiatrist who has treated depressed patients. (See the appendix for how to find a nutritionally oriented doctor.)

Eating Habits

If you have a down day a few times a year, consider whether it might have been precipitated by overindulging in sweets or alcohol. This type of pattern is common between November and January, when people tend to eat too many sugary foods or drink too much alcohol.

Psychological Tips

Have psychological feelings or life experiences contributed to your down days? Sometimes these psychosocial influences are not always obvious. For example, you may feel let down after holiday celebrations, after not getting a promotion or a raise you had hoped for, or even after a vacation when you have to resume more routine activities.

It may help to simply take the day off work and do something you might otherwise do on a weekend. Some people call these "psychological sick days"—when they need one extra day away from work. You could spend that day talking with close friends, going window shopping, visiting the zoo or a museum, or taking yourself out to lunch or dinner.

Helpful Supplements

If you wake up feeling down but have to be sharp for work, you might benefit from a simple, natural mood brightener that consists of the amino acid L-tyrosine and vitamin B12. L-tyrosine is needed to make epinephrine and dopamine, neurotransmitters that promote upbeat moods, wakefulness, and feelings of excitement.

Take 500 to 1,000 mg of L-tyrosine about thirty minutes before consuming anything in the morning other than water. Follow this by immediately taking a sublingual (under the tongue) vitamin B12 tablet. TwinLab's 5,000 mcg B-12 Dot product works well for this purpose. Your down feeling should clear after a couple of hours.

Mild, Moderate, and Other Forms of Depression

Depression is a serious feeling of being down that lasts for two or more weeks. If you're depressed, you might describe yourself as being down in the dumps, discouraged, hopeless, sad, or trapped (such as in a bad job or relationship). Doctors use standardized questionnaires to help score the seriousness of a patient's depression, usually rating it as mild, moderate, or major (severe). Dysthymia is a mild form of depression, but one that has lasted for at least two years. Major depression is extremely serious, is difficult to treat, and often involves thoughts about death or suicide. Irritability, constant anger, and angry outbursts may also be signs of depression.

What You Should Know

Depression is characterized by several qualities, some of which might strike you as being obvious and others that indirectly point to the disorder. Among these qualities are

- Feelings of sadness, hopelessness, and pessimism, as well as a lack of motivation, most of the day and almost every day
- Significantly reduced interest or pleasure in activities that were previously enjoyable
- Feelings of worthlessness and low self-esteem
- A sense of guilt
- Fatigue, lack of energy, or sluggishness
- Significant weight gain or weight loss (when not dieting)
- Sleep disturbances, particularly insomnia or lack of restful sleep
- Irritability, worry, anger, or agitation
- Difficulty concentrating or making decisions
- Thinking about or fantasizing about death or suicide

Doctors usually diagnose major depression when at least several of the previous qualities are present. In general, women are far more likely than men to feel depressed. Drug therapies and counseling have limited benefits for both men and women. One-third of patients recover through such therapies, and another third continue to have at least some symptoms. The remaining third don't benefit at all from medications or counseling.

Why do conventional therapies produce such dismal results in depression? They fail to correct underlying nutritional and biochemical problems. For example, a drug that maintains high brain levels of serotonin can work only if a patient is capable of making adequate amounts of the neurotransmitter. Serotonin production depends on protein and vitamin intake, so eating more protein and vegetables (and fewer sugars and refined carbohydrates) is essential for improving moods.

Sometimes the psychosocial aspects of a person's life can create a feeling of utter hopelessness, leading to profound depression. That was the case with Ruth, a devout Catholic who married young and was in an abusive marriage for more than twenty years. With two small boys to care for, she saw no way out of the marriage short of hell, excommunication, or suicide. Because of her predicament, she became an alcoholic and even attempted suicide. On her own, she began to piece together the "Get aware, get willing, and get with it" steps I described earlier. She came to understand her path in life and how to change it into a more positive direction. She sought professional help, joined Alcoholics Anonymous and stopped drinking, got divorced, and went to college and earned a degree.

Some people have a genetic predisposition toward developing chronic depression, especially after experiencing a major life event, such as the death of a loved one. These genetic tendencies reduce the body's ability to either make or transport serotonin, although they can often be corrected with B-vitamin or 5-HTP supplementation. (See the supplement recommendations in the following pages.)

Low thyroid activity might also be a factor in depression, especially if you are a woman and even more so if you are a woman over forty-five years of age. Occasionally, thyroid test results will look normal, but the hormone levels are actually low for you as an individual. Possible clues to low thyroid activity are a lack of energy and not sweating. If you feel that low thyroid might be a factor, and the tests look normal, ask your doctor for a trial prescription of Armour brand thyroid (the most natural of several thyroid medications). If your depression was related to low thyroid, you may feel better within hours or days.

Many medications can predispose people to depression. These drugs include but are not limited to Glucophage and Prilosec, cortisone, estrogen, progesterone, diuretics, L-dopa, barbiturates, and amphetamines. Antidepressant drugs, such as Prozac and Zoloft, can cause a variety of serious side effects. Some adults and children taking these drugs become suicidal. Up to one-half of patients taking these drugs suffer from low sexual libido or performance, a side effect that can be depressing in its own right.

Eating Habits

First, rule out food allergies (discussed in chapter 3). Although dairy- and wheat-containing foods are the most common allergens, any food could be problematic. The food you tend to crave the most is a likely allergen.

Second, follow the dietary guidelines described in chapter 5, emphasizing healthful proteins and a variety of vegetables. Reduce or eliminate refined sugars and carbohydrates because the blood sugar swings they engender can affect your mood.

Psychological Tips

Many therapies can help to reduce feelings of depression, and combining them with dietary changes and nutritional supplements will improve your chances of recovery.

Redirect your negative self-talk. Depressed people are often very self-critical. When they make a mistake or fail to finish a task, they whip themselves with such negative thoughts as, "I can't do anything right" or "What's wrong with me?" Change your negative self-talk into something positive, such as, "I'm going to take the time to do this right."

Talk therapies. People who feel depressed may be socially isolated, and this isolation can actually contribute to feelings of worthlessness. If you are depressed and have at least one close friend or coworker, ask that person if you could talk with him or her for an hour or two. Talking will relieve you of part of your psychological burden, and it will help you to feel more connected to other people.

Even if you have such a friend, you should also consider professional counseling. In general, an individual therapist has a greater influence on your recovery than any particular type of therapy does. That underscores the importance of finding a therapist with whom you are comfortable (though not necessarily someone who will agree with you all the time). Many communities offer free counseling to people who cannot afford it.

That said, two forms of psychotherapy seem to provide the greatest benefits in easing depression. One is cognitive-behavioral therapy. This approach coaches patients to recognize and consciously correct thought patterns that aggravate symptoms of depression. It often involves homework assignments, such as being more assertive and acting less victim-like at work.

Cognitive-behavioral therapy can also help to deprogram a patient's habits that reinforce feelings of depression. For example, Alyssa suffered from several symptoms of depression, including poor self-esteem. She was especially sensitive to innocent joking comments from friends. On one occasion, the husband of a friend commented that she had an "artist's car"—a vehicle that had seen better days. Alyssa said nothing but drove home feeling that she was a total failure because she couldn't afford a newer car. Eventually, in therapy, she was able to create a more positive self-perception.

A second helpful therapy is called interpersonal therapy. This approach focuses on a patient's difficulties with others. It's particularly helpful with major life transitions, such as a divorce or the death of a spouse, and afterward redefining a relationship with children. Therapy focuses on helping the patient better adapt to the inevitable changes in life.

Exercise. Many studies have found that a regular program of exercise helps to reduce the severity of depression. How does exercise help? Some researchers believe that exercise increases levels of endorphins, a family of natural uppers made by the body. Joggers often refer to a runner's high that is felt after running for a mile or two, and going for a walk can lift feelings of depression for about an hour. Exercise may help for other reasons, too. Regular physical activity adds structure to a person's life, and people with depression often lose some of the organizing structure of their lives. Exercise also increases muscle mass, which improves blood sugar and insulin levels.

Get a pet. It's often difficult for depressed people to make new friends and expand their social support networks. Yet pets are accepting of people who are depressed, seriously ill with cancer, or healthy. Having a pet helps you to create a bond with another living creature, and the benefits are often described as "miraculous." Dogs especially are social creatures and, when treated with kindness, return loyalty, affection, and playfulness.

Helpful Supplements

Many supplements described in this section help to elevate levels of serotonin, a mood-enhancing neurotransmitter. Some of the supplements boost levels of other neurotransmitters, such as dopamine, norepinephrine, and phenylethylamine, which may also have antidepressant benefits. All of these supplements will have collateral benefits because they further a wide range of normal biochemical activities.

High-potency vitamins. Although I frequently recommend a high-potency multivitamin or B-complex vitamin supplement, you might find such supplements of greater benefit in depression if they contain pyridoxyl-5-phosphate, the more biologically active form of vitamin B6. (You'll have to look at the fine print on the label where the ingredients are listed.) If you cannot find a multivitamin or a B-complex supplement with pyridoxyl-5-phosphate, take an additional 50 mg along with your regular supplement. In addition, I recommend that you take the high-potency multivitamin or B-complex supplement for at least two weeks before trying other supplements. The reason is that the B-complex supplement alone may be beneficial, saving you money.

Antidepressant formulas. Many vitamin companies market specific supplements for easing depression, although the labels can legally only hint at this use. One of the best-formulated products is Deproloft, made by Thorne Research (for more information or to order, visit www.thorne.com or call 208-263-1337). It contains several key B vitamins, plus amino acids and herbs. Follow the label directions for use.

SAMe. The body makes S-adenosylmethionine from B vitamins and the amino acid methionine and then puts SAMe to use in making serotonin and other neurotransmitters. As supplements go, SAMe is fairly expensive, but it may boost the effectiveness of B vitamins. By itself, SAMe often works as well as some antidepressant medications, such as imipramine, but it also enhances the benefits of medications in treating major depression (the most severe type). Take 800 to 1,600 mg daily. SAMe may be of particular help if you suffer from both osteoarthritis and depression.

Chromium. This essential dietary mineral plays a crucial role in regulating blood sugar levels and insulin function. If feelings of depression are associated with excessive appetite, overeating, or overweight, supplements of chromium picolinate may be of particular benefit. The discovery of chromium's value in atypical depression was first published in 1999 by Malcolm McLeod, M.D., a psychiatrist at the University of North Carolina School of Medicine, Chapel Hill. Since then, further studies by McLeod and others have confirmed the effectiveness of chromium picolinate in depression that involves overeating. Take 400 mcg daily or 200 mcg twice daily with meals.

5-HTP. Technically known as 5-hydroxytryptophan, 5-HTP is the immediate precursor to serotonin. The supplement increases serotonin levels, whereas antidepressant drugs try to maintain higher levels (which may be difficult if there is not much serotonin to work with). The 5-HTP molecule is built around tryptophan, an amino acid found in meats, fowl, and fish. Pure tryptophan is more difficult to find (to order, visit www.nokomisnutrition.com), but it may actually work a little better, because the body can use tryptophan in a wider range of biochemical reactions. Take 50 to 200 mg of 5-HTP daily, in divided doses, at least one hour prior to or after eating food. For tryptophan, take 500 to 6,000 mg daily, in divided doses, also at least one hour prior to or after eating food. If insomnia is associated with depression, take the last dose thirty minutes before bed.

St. John's wort. Of all the herbal remedies on the market, St. John's wort has the most substantial scientific research behind it. In Europe, the herb is often the first choice for treating mild to moderate depression, as well as dysthymia. Studies have repeatedly shown that St. John's wort works better than the leading prescription drugs, including Prozac, Zoloft, Paxil, and imipramine, and that it also poses fewer side effects than the drugs.

Nutritionally oriented practitioners usually reserve St. John's wort for treating mild to moderate depression but not major depression. Major depression is difficult to treat with any therapy, and, not surprisingly, one study questioned the herb's benefits in severe depression. Another study, however, found that very high doses of the herb were helpful.

St. John's wort can also relieve many of the mood and behavioral symptoms associated with premenstrual syndrome. In one study, virtually all PMS symptoms decreased, with the greatest improvements in anxiety, depression, nervous tension, confusion, and crying.

Take 300 mg of a standardized extract of St. John's wort (such as Carlson Laboratories' St. John's wort, Nature's Way's St. John's wort, or Lichtwer Pharma's Kira product) three times a day. You can also take a comparable tincture (such as A. Vogel Bioforce's Hypericum Tincture). If you suffer from major depression, double the dose.

Note: In serious or long-lasting cases of depression, work with your physician. Do not transition from an antidepressant medication to St. John's wort, and do not combine St. John's wort with antidepressant medications without guidance from your physician.

Omega-3 fish oils. Several studies have found that fish oil supplements may help in depression. These oils are rich in eicosapentaenoic acid (EPA) and docosahexaenoic acid (DHA), members of a family of healthy and essential fats. The contemporary diet is very low in these fats; this allows less healthy fats to take their place and affect brain chemistry. Try 1 to 6 grams daily.

DHEA. The hormone dehydroepiandrosterone is the precursor to estrogen and testosterone. In the 1990s, it became a popular supplement because it often boosted energy levels, increased muscle, and improved libido and sexual performance. In a recent study, researchers used large amounts of DHEA to successfully treat middle-aged men and women with major depression. The subjects also had increases in sexual activity.

Unlike most hormones, DHEA is sold over the counter and is widely available at health food stores and pharmacies. There is great potential for DHEA to be abused, though. You probably don't need DHEA if you are under thirty-five years of age, and odds are that you won't need it if you're younger than fifty. Before taking it, ask your physician to measure your DHEA-S levels. If your DHEA-S levels are low, take 50 to 90 mg of DHEA daily but only under your doctor's supervision. Take larger amounts only if your doctor recommends that you do so, and be sure to have him or her retest your DHEA-S levels after six months and one year.

Quick Tip

Seasonal Affective Disorder

Many people become depressed during the shorter daylight hours of fall and winter, rebounding emotionally during the spring and the summer. This pattern of depression is called seasonal affective disorder, and many researchers believe it is caused by an imbalance in levels of melatonin. This hormone, made by the pineal gland, regulates our circadian, or daily, rhythm and also makes us sleepy. Levels of melatonin tend to increase in the evening, decrease toward morning, and decrease further when we expose ourselves to sunlight. Sunlight suppresses the production of melatonin.

When it's cloudy, when we spend too much time indoors, or when we commute to and from work in the darker days of fall and winter, we're less likely to dispose of our excess melatonin. As a result, our circadian rhythm gets out of kilter, and we tend to feel depressed or physically sluggish.

There are several ways to rectify the problem and reset our circadian clocks. The simplest and cheapest is to spend at least fifteen minutes in the early morning sunlight, such as by going for a walk. If this isn't an easy option, you can take two other steps.

One is to buy a bright full-spectrum lamp or light box (which mimics the full light spectrum of natural daylight) and spend at least fifteen minutes early in the morning reading or working in front of the light. For example, I read my newspapers under a full-spectrum lamp immediately after waking up, and I feel that doing so helps to sharpen my mind.

Another option is to take melatonin supplements, which are sold without a prescription at most health food stores and pharmacies. You'll have to experiment with the dosage—too little won't help and too much may leave you feeling drowsy. Start with a low dose, such as 250 to 500 mcg (0.25 to 0.5 mg), about one to two hours before you go to bed. Don't drive until you get a sense of how drowsy melatonin makes you, and don't combine it with alcohol or any other sedatives. If your initial dose has no effect, increase it to 1 mg and then keep increasing it by 1 mg up to when it starts to have an effect or to a maximum of 9 mg.

It might strike you as odd to take melatonin when you already feel depressed or sluggish. The key is in the timing, which will help you to get a good night's sleep and reset your circadian clock. Even if you're not depressed, melatonin may help if you have difficulty sleeping.

L-Tyrosine. This amino acid is needed to make norepinephrine, epinephrine, and dopamine, all of which are neurotransmitters that are involved in promoting upbeat moods, wakefulness, and feelings of excitement. It is also used in the manufacture of thyroid hormones. L-tyrosine can be a potent natural upper, and you may benefit from daily doses ranging from 500 to 2,000 mg divided in three or four doses each day. L-tyrosine may increase blood pressure, however, so if you have hypertension, please check with your doctor before taking it.

Phenylalanine. If you notice a slight improvement from L-tyrosine but not as much as you would like, try adding 500 mg daily of L-phenylalanine. This is another natural "upper" amino acid and one that the body uses to make L-tyrosine. If you aren't helped by phenylalanine, do not continue to take it. Of course, if you experience a negative reaction to it, stop taking it immediately.

The Ups and Downs of Bipolar Disorder

Bipolar disorder and manic depression are the same mood disorder. Manic depression is still an apt description, but psychiatrists now use the term *bipolar* to describe the same symptoms. Bipolar disorder is generally characterized by alternating episodes of extreme emotional lows (depression) and abnormal mood elevations (mania). The mania can be so intense that people seem to be high or acting like maniacs. Each up or down episode typically lasts from one week to several weeks.

What You Should Know

The main feature of bipolar disorder is the shift between days or weeks of depression to days and weeks of abnormal euphoria. In general, bipolar patients have symptoms of depression about one-third of the time. The manic symptoms consist of repeated episodes of extreme euphoria or irritability, nonstop talking, talking extremely fast, racing thoughts, engaging in risky or dangerous behavior, and going with little or no sleep for days or weeks at a time. The risky behavior comes from a feeling of invulnerability and may affect personal relationships, finances, and business dealings. The odds of having bipolar disorder at some point in your life are surprisingly high—almost 10 percent, according to an article in the *Journal of the American Medical Association.*

Hypomania is a mild form of mania in which people might feel that they are functioning exceptionally well and are especially productive. Some people in the manic phase might say they are "busy with projects" and can't afford to sleep. In such cases, it is usually family members or friends who notice that the person's behavior is unusual or extreme. Hypomania can turn into severe mania, and occasionally, mania will involve psychotic perceptions, including delusions and hallucinations. For example, delusions of grandeur and paranoia may characterize some cases of mania.

At its essence, bipolar disorder reflects a highly unstable brain chemistry. It can develop at any age, but most cases begin during adolescence. The formal diagnosis of bipolar disorder is complicated, and there are several subtypes. Occasionally, the mania form may be misdiagnosed as schizophrenia. Stress, particularly early-life stresses, such as physical or sexual abuse, seems to increase the risk of bipolar disorder.

If you or someone close to you has symptoms of bipolar disorder, it's important to seek treatment by a psychiatrist, at least to stabilize or moderate moods. Lithium is by far the single most effective drug treatment for bipolar disorder; however, it has a narrow effective dose (which will vary from person to person). Too much lithium can cause diarrhea, excessive urination, tremor, and weight gain, and overdoses can be fatal. Valproate (or valproic acid), an anticonvulsant drug, is also used to treat bipolar disorder. But valproate interferes with the body's use of carnitine, an important nutrient, and may result in extreme fatigue.

While these drugs may help to stabilize symptoms, they don't treat the underlying causes of bipolar disorder. Nutrition may further help to reduce symptoms, although it is unlikely to result in a cure.

Eating Habits

Follow the dietary advice described in chapter 5, with a particular emphasis on eating coldwater fish (such as salmon, sardines, and mackerel), which are high in omega-3 fats. These fats are needed for normal brain development and function. Indeed, the high incidence of bipolar

disorder in teenagers might reflect inadequate brain development resulting from a low intake of fish oil.

Psychological Tips

People with bipolar disorder will benefit from a stable home and work
environment. Watchful family members and friends can help by recognizing down-shifting and up-shifting moods in a person with bipolar disorder, leading to better tailoring of medications. Calming activities, such
as those described in chapter 7, may be helpful.

Helpful Supplements

Omega-3 fish oils. Although bipolar disorder is difficult to treat, many
cases seem to respond to omega-3 fish oils, especially those that contain
high levels of eicosapentaenoic acid (EPA). Andrew Stoll, M.D., of the
Harvard Medical School, and his colleagues have found that high doses
of fish oils, such as about 6 grams daily of EPA and 3 grams daily of
docosahexaenoic acid (DHA), are helpful in treating bipolar disorder.
His findings are consistent with other research determining that omega-
3 fish oils benefit a variety of behavioral disorders, including schizophrenia and attention-deficit hyperactivity disorder.

High EPA levels in particular seem useful in treating bipolar disorder,
and Stoll is the codeveloper of Omega-Brite, a fish oil supplement that
contains 90 percent EPA. (Most supplements contain 50 to 65 percent
EPA.) The amount of EPA, however, may be more significant than the
ratio of EPA to DHA, so you may benefit equally from Carlson Laboratories' fish oil capsules or lemon-flavored liquid fish oil.

For bipolar disorder, consider taking 5 to 15 grams of EPA daily—
that's the dose of EPA, not the total amount of oils in the capsules. Start
with the lower dose and increase it gradually over several weeks.
Although the dosage may seem high (and may involve swallowing a lot
of capsules or teaspoons of fish oil), traditional diets in Arctic regions
provide 15 to 19 grams of fish oils daily.

Note: Very high doses of fish oil will have a blood-thinning effect,
which your doctor should monitor if you are taking blood-thinning medications.

High-potency multivitamins. A Canadian study found that a proprietary multivitamin-multimineral supplement may reduce symptoms of bipolar disorder. The formulation, called E M Power + (EMP, or "empower plus"), originated as a veterinary product to calm agitated farm animals; however, clinical testing of the product by doctors at the University of Calgary, Canada, found it helpful in young and middle-aged bipolar patients.

EMP is currently manufactured by Synergy Group of Canada (to order, call 888-878-3467), and the instructions for its use call for taking eight capsules four times a day—a total of thirty-two capsules daily, which may discourage some people. Although the formulation is different from other high-potency vitamin-mineral supplements, a generic supplement may also provide benefits.

Note: EMP and fish oil capsules may potentiate the effect of medications used in the treatment of bipolar disorder. Please work with your physician, who may have to decrease medication doses after you start taking supplements.

13

Dealing with Alcohol and Drug Abuse

One contradiction of our society is that we love alcohol but usually disdain people who abuse it. Less contradictory is the view of drug abuse: nearly everyone in mainstream society sees illegal (street) drugs, such as cocaine and methamphetamine, as being nothing less than addictive and dangerous. Both alcohol and street drugs, regardless of the amount used, alter mood and behavior.

Nutritional deficiencies and imbalances may make some people more susceptible to addictions and related mood issues. Once an addiction is established, it can lead to far more devastating nutrition and health problems.

How prevalent is alcohol and drug abuse? Statistics are little more than educated guesses. Somewhere between eight and thirty million people in the United States abuse alcohol. Almost two million Canadians and three and a half million British are alcohol abusers. Some four to thirteen million people in the United States are believed to be drug abusers. In Canada, the best estimates are that about half a million people regularly abuse drugs, and in Britain, the number is about one million.

How Alcohol and Drugs Affect Mood and Behavior

Nearly everyone is familiar with how alcohol can affect moods and behavior. A small amount, such as a glass of wine or beer, can produce an enjoyable, relaxing effect and can take the edge off a stressful day. A little more can markedly reduce inhibitions, making a person talkative or more interested in having sex. A large amount of alcohol can interfere with male sexual performance, slow reflexes and impair driving, turn intelligent conversation into slurred words and disconnected thoughts, and have a mood-depressing effect. In some people, alcohol's inhibition-reducing effect can set the stage for angry outbursts and physical violence.

Similarly, street drugs can cause a wide variety of mood and behavior changes when a person is either high or going through withdrawal. These changes are usually more extreme than those that occur with alcohol, and they can include euphoria, hallucinations, depression, and mania. Among the many street drugs, cocaine and methamphetamine (meth) are powerful stimulants, and meth is extremely addictive.

Addictions are a form of self-destructive behavior. They entail psychological, neurochemical, and physical dependencies—obsessions, cravings, and the feeling that it's impossible to live without alcohol or drugs. Withdrawal symptoms become uncomfortable and intense, and the addiction begins as a way to avoid withdrawal symptoms. Once the addiction is established, withdrawal becomes painful and difficult. Because alcohol and drugs are costly, addicts often lie to family and friends, cheat, steal, and destroy themselves financially to maintain their addictions.

More Fundamental Effects on Mood and Behavior

Alcohol and drugs modify the body's normal biochemical activities in fundamental and far-reaching ways. For example, alcohol causes more than transient intoxication. Researchers have found that drinking alcohol changes the activity of almost two hundred genes in brain cells. Many of these genes play a role in judgment and decision making, and at least some of these changes could permanently alter gene activity and affect mood and thinking processes.

Cocaine and meth mimic neurotransmitters and radically alter neurotransmitter levels. Cocaine blocks the normal breakdown of dopamine, leading to high levels of the stimulating neurotransmitter. Similarly, meth acts like a super-dopamine and also reduces serotonin transport in the brain by at least half. With high dopamine and low serotonin activity, it's impossible to feel calm.

Long-term, the abuse of alcohol and street drugs results in a variety of health problems. Alcohol stresses the liver and can increase the risk of fatty liver, cirrhosis, and liver cancer. Cocaine and meth can cause blurred vision, seizures, brain damage, heart attacks, fatal kidney and lung diseases, coma, and sudden death.

How Do Addictions Begin?

We live in a drug-oriented society, where pills are routinely sold, prescribed, and assumed to solve our problems, from heartburn to erectile dysfunction. Little wonder, then, that many people are easily lured into abusing alcohol, street drugs, and prescription medicines.

In the United States and many other countries, advertising links alcohol with fun, parties, attractive people, and sex, persuading us that alcohol can make everything in life better. In Ireland, Guinness beer ads weave alcohol into the nation's character with such advertising slogans as "It's Part of Who We Are." Still other types of advertising around the world associate alcohol with sophistication, sports, and being one of the guys.

Between 2001 and 2004, in the United States alone, the makers of alcoholic drinks spent almost $3.5 billion on television advertising and almost $1.5 billion on magazine advertising. Much of the advertising is directed at young adults who often lack judgment about alcohol abuse and the risks of addiction.

People start drinking and continue for many other reasons. One is peer pressure—most people want to fit in socially, and alcohol is a social beverage that erases tensions. It can help us relax, cope with stress, be less inhibited, and reduce physical pain from injuries or disease. For many people, drinking alcohol becomes a central part of their social activities.

Peer pressure often factors in with the use of cocaine, meth, and other street drugs. It's cool and daring to use drugs for the first time, but the initial mental alertness and decreased appetite attract people as well. In a world that values multitasking and increased productivity, the short-term effects of cocaine can be exhilarating. So can be the weight loss that comes from how the drugs suppress appetite.

Like cocaine, meth initially creates a sense of well-being, but regular use quickly leads to aggressive, paranoid, and violent behavior. Meth is broken down much more slowly than cocaine is in the body, and meth users may go up to two weeks without sleeping. They often don't need a provocation to become violent, but confronting a meth user (as police may do) can increase the likelihood of a violent response. When alcohol is combined with meth, the behavior becomes especially volatile. The severe physical consequences of meth, such as premature aging and rotting teeth, are caused by severe nutritional deficiencies (the result of addicts' not eating), but they may also be related to how the drug's activity depletes nutrients.

Denial of an Addiction Problem

Alcoholics and drug addicts often deny they have a problem with substance abuse. Denial is a powerful, self-protective feeling, and people rationalize their addictions in a multitude of ways. People may refuse to admit they have a problem because of the sheer power that addiction has over their lives, the shame and the guilt often associated with alcohol and drug abuse, and the difficulty of changing personal habits. If someone can't acknowledge that a problem exists, it's impossible to begin to recover.

Often, alcoholics and drug abusers sincerely believe they don't have an addiction problem. They may say they only occasionally use alcohol or drugs, or they may argue that they aren't hurting anyone else. The telltale clues are that they have difficulty abstaining, they frequently think about their next opportunity to use alcohol or drugs, or they start to have withdrawal symptoms. If they are alcoholics, they almost always have alcohol at home, often hide it from others, and mix stronger drinks for themselves than for other people.

How, then, does a person accept the fact that he or she has a problem with alcohol or drugs? It's not easy, given the fact that only an estimated 4 percent of alcoholics join Alcoholics Anonymous. To overcome denial, people must own up to what they are doing, such as lying about drinking. There's no surefire way to recognize and overcome denial, but several steps have been known to help. Among them is recognizing that you (if you are an alcoholic or an addict) are hurting the people around you, if not physically, then mentally and emotionally.

Sometimes other people can prompt someone to deal with his or her addiction. An alcoholic or an abuser arrested for driving under the influence may be ordered by the court to go into treatment. Similarly, family members of alcoholics and addicts might try to intervene. Although the alcoholic or the drug abuser denies that he or she has a problem, denial becomes more difficult when a spouse, an employer, a minister, and friends as a group confront that person.

Questions to Ask Yourself

John A. Ewing, M.D., the founding director of the Bowles Center for Alcohol Studies, University of North Carolina, Chapel Hill, developed the four-question CAGE test as a way for physicians to inquire about alcohol abuse in a nonthreatening manner. Two or more "yes" answers suggest a problem with alcohol abuse and justify further inquiry.

You can use this short questionnaire to gauge your risk of alcoholism or adapt it to evaluating a family member.

1. Have you ever felt that you needed to **c**ut down on your drinking?
2. Have people **a**nnoyed you by criticizing your drinking?
3. Have you ever felt **g**uilty about drinking?
4. Have you ever felt that you needed a drink first thing in the morning (an **e**ye-opener) to steady your nerves or get rid of a hangover?

Codependent and Enabling Relationships

Living with, dating, or working with an alcoholic or a drug abuser can create unhealthy enabling or codependent relationships. Enablers encourage or allow people to abuse alcohol and drugs without negative consequences. They may do this passively by not challenging the self-destructive behavior, or they may do it actively by buying alcohol or drugs. Enablers may also protect abusers from the consequences of their actions, such as by making excuses for their moods or behavior.

Melody Beattie, the author of two classic books, *Codependent No More* and *Beyond Codependency*, describes a codependent as a person who either is obsessed with controlling a substance abuser or feels emotionally tormented by continued interactions with him or her. (Codependent relationships may not even involve alcohol or drug abuse. They can be emotionally codependent, which is often the case when one person has a volatile, demanding, or abusive personality.) What motivates the enabler and the codependent? It is often a desire to avoid arguments and conflict, and sometimes it is financial or emotional dependence on the other person.

Therapists and support groups, such as Al-Anon, remind enablers and codependents that they did not cause the addiction and they cannot cure it. Through therapy or interactions in support groups, Al-Anon members learn that they can change only themselves, not the alcoholic or the addict.

Psychological Tips

People seem to either love or hate Alcoholics Anonymous's 12-step recovery program, but there's no denying that it has helped millions of people. The program involves surrendering oneself to a higher authority, usually God, as a central part of its recovery plan. I have known many AA members who have successfully abstained from alcohol for many years. A similar program for drug addicts is called Narcotics Anonymous.

I believe the odds of long-term recovery can be greatly improved by including dietary modification and supplements. (More further on.) In fact, Bill Wilson, the founder of AA, advocated the use of high-potency B vitamins in treating alcoholism.

Can an alcoholic ever go back to drinking in moderation? It's a controversial idea. AA contends that a person who is an alcoholic will always be an alcoholic and should never again drink alcohol. While it's possible that a few people can learn to limit their alcohol intake, the danger is that even small amounts of alcohol may reignite the biochemical and neurochemical basis of addiction in susceptible people. If you have been in recovery, my recommendation is that you stay in recovery.

Because alcohol is often associated with memories of good times, various experiences may trigger a sudden desire for alcohol. Robert, a member of AA, told the story of enjoying a beautiful warm spring day. He was driving his convertible with the top down and thought to himself, "Wouldn't a couple of beers be absolutely great!" Then he realized it was 7 a.m. and the thought was a flashback to when he was drinking years earlier. He immediately banished the thought from his mind.

If you are a social alcoholic, you may have to find new friends after you stop drinking. Alcoholics and drug addicts don't usually like to socialize with people who aren't substance abusers because the nonuser's restraint makes the abuser self-conscious of his or her addiction. Making new friends is often difficult, but AA and NA are often good places to form a new circle of friends, with everyone reinforcing his or her sobriety.

Psychological counseling can be especially helpful, leading to an understanding of how the addiction began and how it affects your life, relationships, and employment. In therapy, people can learn to avoid triggers that might renew alcohol or drug cravings.

Eating Habits

I once interviewed Bill Dufty, the author of *Sugar Blues* and a former musician in Billie Holiday's band. Holiday was an exceptionally talented singer and, sadly, an alcoholic. (She was portrayed by Diana Ross in the movie *Lady Sings the Blues*.) Dufty was with Holiday as she lay on her deathbed, and he noted that she asked not for alcohol but for a soft drink. Years later, he realized that Holiday's addiction to sugar was the underpinning of her addiction to alcohol.

Alcoholism is a form of glucose intolerance, related to the same blood sugar problems that cause diabetes. It's uncertain whether a diet high in sugars and refined carbohydrates causes alcoholism, but such eating habits certainly contribute to it. Because sugars and refined carbohydrates can produce both cravings and withdrawal-like symptoms, they may form a parallel addiction that encourages alcohol abuse.

My dietary recommendations, described in chapter 5, are to eat a protein- and vegetable-rich diet that's low in carbohydrates and sugars. In addition, avoid sugary soft drinks, snacks, and desserts. When snacking, opt for protein or complex carbohydrates, such as a piece of cheese (assuming that you don't have dairy sensitivities) or mixed nuts. Following these guidelines will help to stabilize your blood sugar levels and may decrease alcohol cravings. Better control of blood sugar levels will also result in less stress to the liver, which (with the pancreas) plays a central role in regulating blood sugar levels in the body.

Allergylike food sensitivities may also play a role in alcoholism, particularly in people who prefer a certain type of alcohol. For example, most beers are made from wheat, vodka from rye and other grains, rum from sugar, and bourbon from corn. Cravings for particular types of alcohol suggest related food sensitivities, and it may be wise to avoid those foods as a way to reduce alcohol cravings. In addition, alcohol increases the permeability of the gut, allowing undigested proteins to enter the bloodstream and set off an allergylike immune response.

Although cocaine and meth act via different mechanisms in the body, a similar protein- and vegetable-rich diet will likely be of benefit.

Helpful Supplements

While supplements by themselves are not a cure for alcoholism or drug abuse, they can help to correct biochemistry and reduce cravings. They are best used in combination with other recovery programs and therapies, including better eating habits, counseling, and AA meetings.

Supplements for Alcoholism and Alcohol Abuse

B-complex. A high-potency B-complex supplement can help to restore normal liver function and may help to ease cravings. Look for a supplement containing at least 50 mg each of vitamins B1, B2, and B3. *Note*: Ask your doctor for an injection of B-complex vitamins, which may quickly reduce the desire for alcohol.

Vitamin B1. Consider adding 100 mg extra of vitamin B1 daily because of alcohol-related depletion.

Vitamin B3. Consider adding 1,000 to 2,000 mg of niacinamide daily. *Note*: The niacin form of vitamin B3 causes a flushing sensation that lasts about one hour. Niacinamide does not cause this flush.

Silymarin. This antioxidant extract of the herb milk thistle helps liver function, which may be impaired after long-term alcohol abuse. Take 100 to 300 mg daily.

Kudzu. This herb (*Pueraria lobata*) may decrease the desire for alcohol, leading to a reduction in alcohol intake. Take 1,000 mg three times daily.

Chromium picolinate. This supplement can improve glucose tolerance. Take 500 mcg twice daily.

Probiotics. These supplements of "good" bacteria may help to heal alcohol's damage to the gut wall. Follow the label directions for use.

Body Cleanse and Detox. Consider adopting a cleansing/detox regimen. The Whole Body Cleanse kit from Enzymatic Therapy is a two-week supplement program (available at health food stores or by calling 800-783-2286) that can be used up to four times a year. It contains natural laxatives, silymarin, and other ingredients that help to restore gut and liver function.

Supplements for Cocaine or Meth Abuse

Vitamin C. The brain normally has high concentrations of vitamin C, which can protect against the toxic effects of stimulants. High doses of vitamin C may also alter the activity of opiate receptors in the brain, leading to less interest in drugs. Take 1,000 to 3,000 mg daily.

N-acetylcysteine. NAC may help to restore normal brain levels of glutamate, a calming neurotransmitter. Glutamate is also involved in the production of GABA, another calming neurotransmitter. Researchers have found that high doses of NAC (600 mg four times daily) can reduce the desire for cocaine.

DHEA. Some evidence suggests that the hormone dehydroepiandrosterone may lessen cocaine addiction. Ask your physician to test whether your blood levels of DHEA-S are below normal. If they are low to low normal, consider adding 25 to 50 mg of DHEA daily.

5-HTP or L-tryptophan. In early 2006, researchers found that former meth users had approximately one-half the normal number of serotonin transporters in various brain regions associated with physically aggressive behavior. Long-term meth users had even fewer serotonin transporters. It is possible that serotonin-enhancing nutrients, such as 5-HTP and L-tryptophan, might help to seed new serotonin transporters.

Omega-3 fish oils. Studies show that cocaine users have low levels of omega-3 fats. In one study, researchers gave 3 grams daily of omega-3 fish oils or placebos to twenty-four men with a history of substance abuse. After three months, the men taking the fish oil supplements had a significant decrease in anger, which is associated with aggressive behavior. Still other research indicates that omega-3 fish oils protect brain cells from toxins. Take omega-3 fish oil capsules or liquid to achieve approximately 2,000 mg of EPA (eicosapentaenoic acid) daily.

Selenium. Some evidence suggests that selenium may prevent meth-related brain damage. Take 200 to 400 mcg daily.

Alcohol and drug addictions are difficult to treat. A multipronged approach, as described here, may enhance and reinforce recovery. Needless to say, a certain amount of personal vigilance is required to avoid psychological and social situations that might tempt the use of alcohol or drugs.

Some nutritional medicine centers, such as the Pfeiffer Treatment Center and the Health Recovery Center (see appendix), have had great success in treating addictions by customizing nutritional supplements to patients' individual needs. These treatments rely heavily on the use of amino acid supplements. Because of the seriousness of alcohol and drug abuse, I encourage you to work with a nutritionally oriented health care professional.

Afterword

The world is a meaner, angrier, and more anxious place than it was just a few years ago. Regardless of your age, you've been around long enough to witness at least some of these undesirable changes in the form of increased crime, terrorism, or war in the world around us. These changes reflect a world that seems increasingly stressful and in a downward spiral. If you doubt what I write, read the newspaper, watch the news, and ask yourself: Is the world a better, safer, and kinder place than it was five or ten years ago?

I certainly don't blame all of our social problems, from violent crimes to terrorism, on bad eating habits. After all, the way we eat is shaped by our society and influences that include family upbringing, peer pressure, our knowledge about food, the stresses we face, food availability, and the amount of time we have to shop and prepare meals. Eating habits do affect our moods and behavior, however, and in this way they contribute to the tenor of the world. You need look no further than the late-afternoon rush hour to see how hunger and low blood sugar affect our patience on the road. When large numbers of people have bad moods, or powerful people have bad moods, there is a greater risk of negative emotional chain reactions.

You could argue that the human race has always had a violent streak, and you would be right. And I would counter that people have often lived in times of poor or unbalanced diets. When our nutritional intake is marginal, our moods and behavior are likely to be marginal as well. Some people will always be more susceptible than others to the behavioral and physical effects of poor nutrition.

What's even worse, bad nutrition and bad moods are not just a problem in your community or only an American problem. As U.S. companies have increasingly exported their junk foods to other nations, the incidence of obesity and diabetes has soared. I would also argue that so has the preponderance of bad moods. Again, I cannot blame all the world's religious and political strife on bad diets, but it's inevitable that bad diets contribute to some of the seeds of conflict because they interfere with healthy moods and how we think and act.

Unfortunately, you and I are probably not in a position to make sweeping improvements in our cities, our country, or the world. Many other people wield far greater power in politics, eating habits, and economics than we do, and we are no match for the billions of dollars that junk food companies spend on marketing and advertising. Yet we can make a difference as individuals.

How can we do this?

I have long believed that positive, long-lasting social change—characterized by greater patience, tolerance, and fairness—is best accomplished on a grassroots, one-to-one basis. For example, we cannot legislate the eating habits of millions of adults; however, people in many communities have successfully urged their governments to prohibit the sale of junk foods in public schools. It's a small step, one of a great many steps to be taken, but an important step nonetheless.

It's also important that we relearn how to connect with other human beings, to break bread with them. To do this, we must consider what we share in common instead of emphasizing our opposing political, social, and religious views. I believe that improving our moods will help to restore some of the patience we need to talk with and accept people who hold different beliefs. We can learn from one another.

As individuals, we have the power to control our own eating habits and do many other things to improve our moods and behavior, as well as our overall health. Every day presents us with countless opportunities to make important choices. We can choose to drive to a fast-food restaurant for a burger, fries, and a soft drink or go to a market for more healthful and wholesome foods. We can react with irritation and anger at inconsiderate drivers, or we can take a deep breath to protect ourselves against negative emotional shrapnel. Instead of furthering a cascade of bad moods, we can foster good moods. We can influence the eating habits and the lifestyles of our family members and set an example for our friends and coworkers.

And we can, in small ways, affect the quality of foods in the marketplace. Businesses want to earn a profit, and we can dictate the foods they produce by how we spend our money. The phenomenal growth of organic foods is one example. Ten years ago, organic foods were a niche in the health food industry. Today, being organic is a sophisticated and powerful selling point. As another example, a small town in Italy recently rededicated itself to traditional food shops and, in doing so, forced a fast-food restaurant out of business. We can support markets and restaurants that cater to healthful and nutritious foods, and we can encourage other people to do the same.

You have the power to change your life. Every single step you take toward health improves your life, creating gentle ripples that positively affect the people around you. Start taking those steps today. Once you start, you'll never want to stop. You'll feel better and your mind will be clearer, and you'll help to make the world a better place.

APPENDIX

Resources for Supplements, Foods, and Additional Information

Working with a nutritionally oriented physician or psychiatrist can usually help you to identify and improve mood and behavior problems. These organizations provide referral services.

Referral Organizations for Finding Nutritionally Oriented Physicians and Psychiatrists

American College for Advancement in Medicine
www.acam.org

American Association of Naturopathic Physicians
www.naturopathic.org

International Society for Orthomolecular Medicine
www.orthomed.org or centre@orthomed.org

Nutritionally (Biochemically) Oriented Treatment Centers

Bright Spot for Health/Riordan Center *(focusing on mood and degenerative physical diseases)*
3100 N. Hillside Avenue
Wichita, KS 67219
(316) 682-3100

Health Recovery Center *(focusing on mood and behavior)*
3255 Hennepin Avenue South
Minneapolis, MN 55408
(800) 554-9155

Pfeiffer Treatment Center *(focusing on mood and behavior)*
4575 Weaver Parkway
Warrenville, IL 60555-4039
(630) 505-0300
www.hriptc.org

Psychologists and Counselors

You can often get a recommendation for a psychologist or a counselor from your primary care physician or a friend. Because some state standards are lax, inquire whether a specific psychologist or counselor is licensed or certified by the state in which you live. You can also get referrals through these Web sites.

Network Therapy, a Mental Health Network
www.networktherapy.com

Psychology Today magazine referral services
www.psychologytoday.com

Nutritional Supplements

Thousands of companies sell proprietary brands of vitamins, minerals, and other types of nutritional supplements. I've found the companies listed in the following pages to have high-quality and reliable products.

Advanced Physicians' Products
Founded by a nutritionally oriented physician, APP offers an extensive line of high-quality vitamin and mineral supplements. For more information, call (800) 220-7687 or go to www.nutritiononline.com.

alphabetic and Abkit, Inc.
Abkit manufactures and distributes a variety of excellent supplements and cosmetic products. Its alphabetic is a well-rounded once-a-day supplement for people who are prediabetic or who have diabetes. The company's extensive CamoCare line of cosmetics is designed around the venerable antioxidant herb chamomile. For more information, call (800) 226-6227 or go to www.abkit.com or www.alphabetic.com.

Bioforce
Bioforce, also known as A. Vogel, is a venerable Swiss manufacturer of herbal products, with a strong commitment to product consistency and quality. Most of the company's products consist of standardized tinctures. For more information, call (877) 232-6060 or go to www.bioforce.com.

Carlson Laboratories
Carlson Laboratories offers the widest selection of natural vitamin E products, exceptional fish oil supplements, and a broad range of other vitamin and mineral supplements. It is also the manufacturer of Mellow Mood, one of the products I recommend. For more information, call (800) 323-4141 or go to www.carlsonlabs.com.

Insulow

This company sells Insulow, a unique product that combines the more biologically active "R" form of lipoic acid (an antioxidant) with biotin (a B vitamin). This combination of ingredients helps to regulate blood sugar and insulin levels, which is particularly important for people with glucose-tolerance problems, prediabetes, and diabetes. For more information, call (407) 384-3388 or go to www.insulow.com.

Nature's Way

Nature's Way is a leading herb supplement company whose products include many German pharmaceutical-grade herbal supplements. Most of the company's products are in capsule form. For more information, call the company at (801) 489-1500 or go to www.naturesway.com.

Nutricology/Allergy Research Group

Nutricology/Allergy Research Group is often at the cutting edge of original nutritional supplement formulations. Nutricology is the company's consumer brand, and Allergy Research Group is the company's professional (physician's) brand. For more information, call (800) 545-9960 or go to www.nutricology.com.

Nutrition 21

Nutrition 21 is the company behind the popular Chromax brand of chromium picolinate, which is also sold under much more familiar brand names. In addition, Nutrition 21 also sells Chromax and Diachrome, the latter a chromium picolinate/biotin combination.

Thorne Research

Thorne sells its extensive line of high-quality supplements primarily to physicians, but it also accepts orders from consumers. For more information, call (208) 263-1337 or go to www.thorne.com.

Natural Food Grocers

I recommend that you eat nutrient-dense fresh and natural foods. Your best bet for finding meat from range- or grass-fed animals and organic fruits and vegetables is a natural foods or specialty grocery store. Always read the find print on packages to ascertain ingredients.

Trader Joe's

Trader Joe's is a chain of high-quality specialty retail grocery stores, with many organic, gluten-free, and wholesome products. For more information and the locations of Trader Joe's stores, go to www.traderjoes.com.

Vitamin Cottage

This Colorado-based, family-owned group of twenty natural food stores has markets in Denver and other cities in Colorado, as well as in Albuquerque and

Santa Fe, New Mexico. For more information and the locations of Vitamin Cottage stores, call (877) 986-4600 or go to www.vitamincottage.com.

Whole Foods

At Whole Foods, the emphasis is on wholesome, natural foods, including free-range meats, organic produce, and a wide variety of other healthful food products. For more information, go to www.wholefoods.com.

Wild Oats

This national chain emphasizes natural and gourmet foods. Wild Oats' meat departments offer free-range meats. For more information, call (800) 494-WILD or go to www.wildoats.com.

Specialty Foods and Other Products

Blue Diamond Natural

This company makes "Nut-Thins," some of the best snack crackers you'll find, all free of wheat and gluten products. They include almond, hazelnut, pecan, and almond with cheddar cheese Nut-Thins. They're sold at most health and natural food markets. For more information, go to www.bluediamond.com.

CC Pollen

If you exercise regularly and intensely, you may require relatively high-carb energy bars. CC Pollen makes Almond-Date, Cinnamon-Apple, and Peanut-Raisin Buzz Bars, which are among the best-tasting energy bars sold. The principal sweetener in these bars is honey, and they also contain small amounts of bee pollen harvested in southern Arizona. Many health food stores and Web sites sell Buzz Bars. You can also order them directly from CC Pollen by calling (800) 875-0096 or visiting www.ccpollen.com or www. buzzbars.com.

Earth Song Whole Foods

Earth Song makes several whole-grain snack bars that redefine the meaning of a wholesome sweet. Among the bars are apple-walnut and cranberry-orange. In addition, Earth Song blends an excellent gluten-free muesli, known as Grandpa's Secret Omega-3 Muesli, which makes for a tasty and quick breakfast (if you take about five minutes to prepare it the night before). For more information, call (877) 327-8476 or go to www.earthsongwholefoods.com.

Futters Nut Butters

Futters Nut Butters is a small family-owned company that sells organic nut butters. Some of the nut butters are raw and others are dry roasted. In addition to being organic, they are delightfully simple: a jar contains only the nut butter—no other ingredients. Among the options are almond, hazelnut, macadamia, and pistachio nut butters. For more information, call (877) 772-2155 or go to www.futtersnutbutters.com.

Garlic Gold

Rinaldo's Organic Garlic Gold products include several tasty garlic-based items. Among them are Garlic Gold Nuggets, which are toasted garlic pieces that can be substituted for bacon bits, as well as garlic-infused olive oil. For more information, call Seven Oaks Ranch, the maker, at (800) 695-7673 or go to www.garlicgold.com.

Greens8000

One serving of this greens drink provides the antioxidant power of twenty servings of fruits and vegetables. It also tastes great, something rare among similar products. You add one scoop to a glass of water, stir, and drink. Greens8000 is sweetened with stevia and other natural sweeteners (such as spearmint) and contains only 49 calories and 5 grams of carbohydrates per serving. If you have celiac disease, be aware that it may contain trace amounts of gluten (a few parts per million, according to the company), owing to a small amount of barley malt. While Greens8000 shouldn't replace fruits and vegetables in your diet, it's a great way of getting some of the extra nutrients that are found in fruits, vegetables, and herbs. For more information, go to www.greens8000.com.

Lara Bars

Lara Bars use simple, nutritious ingredients, such as dates and nuts, to create some of the best-tasting energy bars on the market. The flavors include Ginger Snap, Apple Pie, and Cashew Cookie. They're sold at many health food stores and at Trader Joe's. For more information, go to www.larabar.com.

Lotus Foods

Lotus Foods sells a variety of original and tasty rice and rice flour products, including Bhutanese Red Rice and purple Forbidden Rice. The rice flours can be used to dredge fish and chicken, as well as to make gluten-free crepes. For more information, call (510) 525-3137 or go to www.lotusfoods.com to order or to find recipes.

MacNut Oil (Macadamia Nut Oil)

MacNut Oil, made from Australian macadamia nuts, is rich in oleic acid, the same type of fat that makes olive oil so healthful. MacNut Oil has a slight nutty flavor and a higher smoke point than olive oil. For information, call (866) 462-2688 or go to www.macnutoil.com.

Monroe Institute

The Monroe Institute researches audio tones and music designed to heighten specific moods or mental states, including mental sharpness and relaxation.

The institute also sells compact disks with these sounds and music. The CDs are not a gimmick—they really do work. To properly use them, you'll need stereo headphones. For more information, visit www.monroeinstitute.org.

Point Reyes Preserves

This small, family-owned business sells some of the best marinated foods (though they're called "pickled" instead of "marinated") in small shops in and around Point Reyes, California, and by mail order. The products include Pickled Asparagus, Pickled Artichoke Hearts, Pickled Mushrooms, Pickled Beets, Pickled Garlic, Pickled Brussels Spouts, Kosher Dill Pickles, Bread and Butter Pickles, and Corn Relish. All of the products are made from family recipes that have been passed down for generations. The vegetables are grown locally, and the products contain no artificial additives or preservatives. For more information, visit www.pointreyespreserves.com; e-mail jevans@horizoncable.com; or write Point Reyes Preserves, P.O. Box 1341, Point Reyes Station, CA 94956.

Terrapin Ridge

Terrapin Ridge makes and sells an extensive line of tasty sauces, such as Apple Dill and Rosemary, Apricot Honey with Tarragon, and Spicy Chipotle Squeeze, as well as fifteen different mustards. If you are tired of the same old chicken, turkey, or beef, these sauces can add bright new flavors to your meals. For more information, call (800) 999-4052 or go to www.terrapinridge.com.

Newsletters, Books, and Web Sites

Many publications provide excellent information on diet and supplements, though you may sometimes have to navigate contradictory information or ignore information that's inconsistent with my dietary and supplement recommendations.

Newsletters and Books

The Nutrition Reporter™. This monthly newsletter, produced by Jack Challem (the author of this book), summarizes recent research on vitamins, minerals, and herbs. The annual subscription rate is $27 ($48 CND for Canada, $38 U.S. funds for all other countries). For a sample issue, send a business-size self-addressed envelope, with postage for two ounces, to The Nutrition Reporter, P.O. Box 30246, Tucson, AZ 85751. Sample issues are also available at www.nutritionreporter.com.

Feed Your Genes Right (John Wiley & Sons, 2005, $14.95), by Jack Challem. This book focuses on how our genes depend on vitamins and other nutrients, and how we can make the most of our inheritance and reduce the risk of disease.

The Inflammation Syndrome: The Complete Nutritional Program to Prevent and Reverse Heart Disease, Arthritis, Diabetes, Allergies, and Asthma (John Wiley & Sons, 2003, $14.95), by Jack Challem. With a diet plan similar to the one in *Feed Your Genes Right*, this book is tailored more to people with chronic inflammatory diseases.

Syndrome X: The Complete Nutritional Program to Prevent and Reverse Insulin Resistance (John Wiley & Sons, 2000, $14.95), by Jack Challem, Burton Berkson, M.D., Ph.D., and Melissa Diane Smith. With a diet program similar to the one in *Feed Your Genes Right*, this book focuses more on preventing diabetes and heart disease, as well as on losing weight.

Web Sites

The Official Anti-Inflammation Diet Plan Web Site
www.inflammationsyndrome.com

Medline/PubMed
The world's largest searchable database of medical journal articles, providing free abstracts (summaries) of more than 8 million articles.
www.pubmed.gov

Merck Manual
The online edition of your physician's standard medical reference book.
www.merck.com

Nutrient Data Laboratory Food Composition
Type in nearly any food or food product, and you instantly get its nutritional breakdown per cup or 100 grams.
www.ars.usda.gov/

The Nutrition Reporter™
Dozens of articles on vitamins and minerals.
www.nutritionreporter.com

The Official No More Bad Moods Web Site
www.foodmoodsolution.com

Price-Pottenger Foundation
A Web site dedicated to two twentieth-century nutritional pioneers.
www.price-pottenger.org

SELECTED REFERENCES

A complete list of references is available at www.foodmoodsolution.com.

Introduction

Grant BF, Stinson FS, Dawson DA, et al. Prevalence and co-occurrence of substance use disorders and independent mood and anxiety disorders. *Archives of General Psychiatry*, 2004;61:807–816.

Kessler RC, Berglund P, Demler O, et al. Lifetime prevalence and age-of-onset distributions of *DMS-IV* disorders in the national comorbidity survey replication. *Archives of General Psychiatry*, 2005;62:593–602.

Zernike K. Violent crimes rising sharply in some cities. An increase in killing over petty disputes. *New York Times*, February 12, 2006:A1.

Chapter 1. How Food Affects Your Mood

Benton D, Haller J, Fordy J. Vitamin supplementation for 1 year improves mood. *Neuropsychobiology*, 1995;32:98–105.

Cassata D. Rude behavior: it's a crass reality across hurried America, poll finds. *Arizona Daily Star* (Associated Press), October 15, 2005:A1.

Gesch CB, Hammond SM, Hampson SE, et al. Influence of supplementary vitamins, minerals, and essential fatty acids on the antisocial behavior of young adult prisoners. *British Journal of Psychiatry*, 2002;181:22–28.

Walsh WJ, Glab LB, Haakenson ML. Reduced violent behavior following biochemical therapy. *Physiology and Behavior*, 2004;82:835–839.

Chapter 2. How Life's Stresses Do a Number on Your Moods

Arnedt JT, Owens J, Crouch M, et al. Neurobehavioral performance of residents after heavy night call vs after alcohol ingestion. *JAMA*, 2005;294:1025–1033.

Ayas NT, White DP, Manson JE, et al. A prospective study of sleep duration and coronary heart disease in women. *Archives of Internal Medicine*, 2003;163:205–209.

Dallman MF, Pecoraro N, Akana SF, et al. Chronic stress and obesity: a new view of "comfort food." *Proceedings of the National Academy of Sciences*, 2003;100:11696–11701.

Dallman MF, Pecoraro NC, la Fleur SE. Chronic stress and comfort foods: self-medication and abdominal obesity. *Brain, Behavior, and Immunity*, 2005;19:275–280.

Hairston IS, Little MT, Scanlon MD, et al. Sleep restriction suppresses neuro-genesis induced by hippocampus-dependent learning. *Journal of Neuro-physiology*, 2005;94:4224–4233.

Hakkarainen R, Johansson C, Kieseppa T, et al. Seasonal changes, sleep length and circadian preference among twins with bipolar disorder. *BMC Psychiatry*, 2003;3:6–12.

Howarth E, Hoffman MS. A multidimensional approach to the relationship between mood and weather. *British Journal of Psychology*, 1984;75(Part 1):12–23.

Keltikangas-Jarvinen L, Raikkonen K, Hautanen A, et al. Vital exhaustion, anger expression, and pituitary and adrenocortical hormones. Implications for the insulin resistance syndrome. *Arteriosclerosis, Thrombosis and Vascular Biology*, 1996;16:275–280.

Kiecolt-Glaser JK, Preacher KJ, MacCallum RC, et al. Chronic stress and age-related increases in the proinflammatory cytokine IL-6. *Proceedings of the National Academy of Sciences*, 2003;100:9090–9095.

Oaten M, Cheng K. Academic examination stress impairs self-control. *Journal of Social and Clinical Psychology*, 2005;24:254–279.

Schory TJ, Piecznski N, Nair S, et al. Barometric pressure, emergency psychiatric visits, and violent acts. *Canadian Journal of Psychiatry*, 2003;48:624–627.

Wertz AT, Wright KP, Ronda JM, et al. Effects of sleep inertia on cognition. *JAMA*, 2006;295:163–164.

Chapter 3. Neuronutrients, Moods, and Your Mind

Cox DJ, Kovatchev BP, Gonder-Frederick LA, et al. Relationships between hyperglycemia and cognitive performance among adults with type 1 and type 2 diabetes. *Diabetes Care*, 2005;28:71–77.

Finger TE, Danilova V, Barrows J, et al. ATP signaling is crucial for communication from taste buds to gustatory nerves. *Science*, 2005;310:1495–1499.

Leventhal AG, Wang Y, Pu M, et al. GABA and its antagonists improved visual cortical function in senescent monkeys. *Science*, 2003;300:812–815.

Chapter 4. The First Step: Take Your Supplements

Alpert JE, Papakostas G, Mischoulon D, et al. S-adenosyl-l-methionine (SAMe) as an adjunct for resistant major depressive disorder. *Journal of Clinical Psychopharmacology*, 2004;24:661–664.

Anonymous. DMG and obsessive-compulsive behaviors. *Autism Research Review International*, 1996;10:7.

Bell C, Abrams J, Nutt D. Tryptophan depletion and its implications for psychiatry. *British Journal of Psychiatry*, 2001;178:399–405.

Benjamin J, Agam G, Levine J, et al. Inositol treatment in psychiatry. *Psychopharmacology Bulletin*, 1995;31:167–175.

Benton D, Fordy J, Haller J. The impact of long-term vitamin supplementation on cognitive functioning. *Psychopharmacology*, 1995;117:298–305.

Benton D, Haller J, Fordy J. Vitamin supplementation for 1 year improves mood. *Neuropsychobiology*, 1995;32:98–105.

Brenner R, Azbel V, Madhusoodanan S, et al. Comparison of an extract of hypericum (LI 160) and sertraline in the treatment of depression: a double-blind, randomized pilot study. *Clinical Therapeutics*, 2000;22:411–419.

Clancy J, Hoffer A, Lucy J, et al. Design and planning in psychiatric research as illustrated by the Weyburn Chronic Nucleotide Project. *Bulletin of the Menninger Clinic*, 1954;18:147–153.

Elmadfa I, Majchrzak D, Rust P, et al. The thiamine status of adult humans depends on carbohydrate intake. *International Journal for Vitamin and Nutrition Research*, 2001;71:217–221.

Eussen SJ, de Groot LC, Clarke R, et al. Oral cyanocobalamin supplementation in older people with vitamin B12 deficiency. *Archives of Internal Medicine*, 2005;165:1167–1172.

Fux M, Levine J, Aviv A, et al. Inositol treatment of obsessive-compulsive disorder. *American Journal of Psychiatry*, 1996;153:1219–1221.

Gannon MC, Nuttall JA, Nuttall FQ. The metabolic response to ingested glycine. *American Journal of Clinical Nutrition*, 2002;76:1302–1307.

Hallahan B, Garland MR. Essential fatty acids and their role in the treatment of impulsivity disorders. *Prostaglandins, Leukotrienes and Essential Fatty Acids*, 2004;71:211–216.

Hamazaki T, Thienprasert A, Kheovichai K, et al. The effect of docosahexaenoic acid on aggression in elderly Thai subjects—a placebo-controlled double-blind study. *Nutritional Neuroscience*, 2002;5:37–41.

Iribarren C, Markovitz JH, Jacobs DR, et al. Dietary intake of n-3, n-6 fatty acids and fish: relationship with hostility in young adults—the CARDIA study. *European Journal of Clinical Nutrition*, 2004;58:24–31.

Kaplan BJ, Fisher JE, Crawford SG, et al. Improved mood and behavior during treatment with a mineral-vitamin supplement: an open label case series of children. *Journal of Child and Adolescent Psychopharmacology*, 2004;14:115–122.

Kennedy DO, Scholley AB, Wesnes KA. The dose-dependent cognitive effects of acute administration of Ginkgo biloba in healthy young volunteers. *Psychopharmacology*, 2000;151:416–423.

Leventhal AG, Wang Y, Pu M, et al. GABA and its antagonists improved visual cortical function in senescent monkeys. *Science*, 2003;300:812–815.

Levine M, Conry-Cantilena C, Wang Y, et al. Vitamin C pharmacokinetics in healthy volunteers: evidence for a recommended dietary allowance. *Proceedings of the National Academy of Sciences*, 1996;93:3704–3709.

Lustman PJ, Anderson RJ, Freedland KE, et al. Depression and poor glycemic control. *Diabetes Care*, 2000;23:934–942.

Mason R. 200 mg of zen: L-theanine boosts alpha waves, promotes alert relaxation. *Alternative and Complementary Therapies*, 2001;7:91–95.

McLeod MN, Golden RN. Chromium treatment of depression. *International Journal of Neuropsychopharmacology*, 2000;3:311–314.

Mousain-Bose M, Roche M, Rapin J, et al. Magnesium vitB6 intake reduces central nervous system hyperexcitability in children. *Journal of the American College of Nutrition*, 2004;23:545S–548S.

Palatnik A, Prolov K, Fux M, et al. Double-blind, controlled crossover trial of inositol versus fluvoxamine for the treatment of panic disorder. *Journal of Clinical Psychopharmacology*, 2001;21:335–339.

Philipp M, Kohnen R, Hiller KO. Hypericum extract versus imipramine or placebo in patients with moderate depression: randomized multicentre study of treatment for eight weeks. *British Medical Journal*, 1999;319:1534–1539.

Schrader E. Equivalence of St. John's wort extract (Ze 117) and fluoxetine: a randomized controlled study in mild-moderate depression. *International Clinical Psychopharmacology*, 2000;15:61–68.

Stevinson C, Ernst E. A pilot study of *Hypericum perforatum* for the treatment of premenstrual syndrome. *British Journal of Obstetrics and Gynaecology*, 2000;107:870–876.

Szegedi A, Kohnen R, Dienel A, et al. Acute treatment of moderate to severe depression with hypericum extract WS 5570 (St. John's wort): randomized controlled double blind non-inferiority trial versus paraxetine. *British Medical Journal*, 2005;330:503–507.

Tildesley NTJ, Kennedy DO, Perry EK, et al. Positive modulation of mood and cognitive performance following administration of acute doses of *Salvia lavandulaefolia* essential oil to healthy young volunteers. *Physiology and Behavior*, 2005;83:699–709.

Wesnes KA, Ward T, McGinty A, et al. The memory enhancing effects of a Ginkgo biloba/Panax ginseng combination in healthy middle-aged volunteers. *Psychopharmacology*, 2000;152:353–361.

Wyatt KM, Simmock PW, Jones PW, et al. Efficacy of vitamin B-6 in the treatment of premenstrual syndrome: systematic review. *British Medical Journal*, 1999;318:1375–1381.

Woelk H, et al. Comparison of St. John's wort and imipramine for treating depression: randomized controlled trial. *British Medical Journal*, 2000;321:536–539.

Chapter 5. The Second Step: Eat Mood-Enhancing Foods

Vander Wal JS, Marth JM, Khosla P, et al. Short-term effect of eggs on satiety in overweight and obese subjects. *Journal of the American College of Nutrition*, 2005;24:510–515.

Chapter 6. The Third Step: Be More Active

Ahlberg AC, Ljung T, Rosmond R, et al. Depression and anxiety symptoms in relation to anthropometry and metabolism in men. *Psychiatry Research*, 2002;112:101–110.

Antunes HK, Stella SG, Santos RF, et al. Depression, anxiety and quality of life scores in seniors after an endurance exercise program. *Revista Brasileira de Psiquiatra*, 2005;27:266–271.

Dunn AL, Trivedi MH, Kampert JB, et al. Exercise treatment for depression: efficacy and dose response. *American Journal of Preventive Medicine*, 2005;28:1–8.

Gaul-Alcacova P, Boucek J, Stejskal P, et al. Assessment of the influence of exercise on heart rate variability in anxiety patients. *Neuro Endocrinology Letters*, December 28, 2005;26:epub ahead of print.

Chapter 7. The Fourth Step: Begin Changing Your Life Habits

Arnedt JT, Wilde GJS, Munt PW, et al. How do prolonged wakefulness and alcohol compare in the decrements they produce on a simulated driving task. *Accident Analysis and Prevention*, 2001;33:337–344.

Berk LS, Tan SA, Fry WF, et al. Neuroendocrine and stress hormone changes during mirthful laughter. *American Journal of Medical Sciences*, 1989;298:390–396.

Kozorovitskiy Y, Gross CG, Kopil C, et al. Experience induces structural and biochemical changes in the adult primate brain. *Proceedings of the National Academy of Sciences*, 2005;102:17478–17482.

Mason R. The sound medicine of Brian Dailey, M.D., F.A.C.E.P. *Journal of Alternative and Complementary Therapies*, 2004;10:156–160.

Rossi EL. Psychosocial genomics: Gene expression, neurogenesis, and human experience in mind-body medicine. *Advances in Body-Mind Medicine*, 2002;18:22–30.

Smyth JM, Stone AA, Hurewitz A, et al. Effects of writing about stressful experiences on symptom reduction in patients with asthma or rheumatoid arthritis: a randomized trial. *JAMA*, 1999;281:1304–1309.

Chapter 8. Dealing with Irritability, Anger, Aggressiveness, and Violent Behavior

Bertone-Johnson ER, Hankinson SE, Bendich A, et al. Calcium and vitamin D intake and risk of incident premenstrual syndrome. *Archives of Internal Medicine*, 2005;165:1246–1252.

Levine M, Conry-Cantilena C, Wang Y, et al. Vitamin C pharmacokinetics in healthy volunteers: evidence for a recommended dietary allowance. *Proceedings of the National Academy of Sciences*, 1996;93:3704–3709.

Sekine Y, Ouchi Y, Takei N, et al. Brain serotonin transporter density and aggression in abstinent methamphetamine abusers. *Archives of General Psychiatry*, 2006;63:90–100.

Walsh WJ, Glab LB, Haakenson ML. Reduced violence behavior following biochemical therapy. *Physiology and Behavior*, 2004;82:835–839.

Wells AS, Read NW, Laugharne JDE, et al. Alterations in mood after changing to a low-fat diet. *British Journal of Nutrition*, 1998;79:23–30.

Chapter 9. Reducing Anxiety, Panic Attacks, and Obsessive-Compulsive Behavior

Atmaca M, Tezcan E, Kuloglu M, et al. Serum folate and homocysteine in patients with obsessive-compulsive disorder. *Psychiatry and Clinical Neurosciences*, 2005;59:616–620.

Benjamin J, Levine J, Fux M, et al. Double-blind, placebo-controlled, crossover trial of inositol treatment for panic disorder. *American Journal of Psychiatry*, 1995;152:1084–1086.

Hughes JR, Higgins ST, Bickel WK, et al. Caffeine self-administration, withdrawal, and adverse effects among coffee drinkers. *Archives of General Psychiatry*, 1991;48:611–617.

Lafleur DL, Pittenger C, Kelmendi B, et al. N-acetylcysteine augmentation in serotonin reuptake inhibitor refractory obsessive-compulsive disorder. *Psychopharmacology*, 2006;184:254–256.

Mills DE, Prkachin KM, Harvey KA, et al. Dietary fatty acid supplementation alters stress reactivity and performance in man. *Journal of Human Hypertension*, 1989;3:111–116.

Pittenger C, Krystal JH, Coric V. Initial evidence of the beneficial effects of glutamate-modulating agents in the treatment of self-injurious behavior associated with borderline personality disorder. *Journal of Clinical Psychiatry*, 2005;66(11):1492–1493.

Prousky JE. Supplemental niacinamide mitigates anxiety symptoms: three case reports. *Journal of Orthomolecular Medicine*, 2005;20:167–178.

Seelig MS, Berger AR, Spielholz N. Latent tetany and anxiety, marginal magnesium deficit, and normocalcemia. *Diseases of the Nervous System*, 1975;36:461–465.

Chapter 10. Reducing Distractible and Impulsive ADHD-like Behavior

Anonymous. Parkinson's drug linked to compulsive behavior. *Arizona Daily Star* (Associated Press), July 12, 2005:A2.

Henig RM. Driving? Maybe you shouldn't be reading this. *New York Times*, July 13, 2005:D5.

Leventhal AG, Wang Y, Pu M, et al. GABA and its antagonists improved visual cortical function in senescent monkeys. *Science*, 2003;300:812–815.

Maayan R, Lotan S, Doron R, et al. Dehydroepiandrosterone (DHEA) attenuates cocaine-seeking behavior in the self-administration model in rats. *European Neuropsychopharmacology*, 2005;16:329–339.

Mousain-Bosc M, Roche M, Rapin J, et al. Magnesium vitB6 intake reduces central nervous system hyperexcitability in children. *Journal of the American College of Nutrition*, 2004;23:545S–548S.

Richardson AJ, Montgomery P. The Oxford-Durham study: a randomized, controlled trial of dietary supplementation with fatty acids in children with developmental coordination disorder. *Pediatrics*, 2005;115:1360–1366.

Saugstad LR. A "new-old" way of thinking about brain disorder, cerebral excitability—the fundamental property of nervous tissue. *Medical Hypotheses*, 2005;64:142–150.

Chapter 11: The Overweight-Prediabetes Connection to Mood Swings

Davidson JR, Abraham K, Connor KM, et al. Effectiveness of chromium in atypical depression: a placebo-controlled trial. *Biological Psychiatry*, 2003;53:261–264.

Khan A, Safdar M, Khan MMA, et al. Cinnamon improves glucose and lipids of people with type 2 diabetes. *Diabetes Care*, 2003; 26:3215–3218.

Kim MS, Park JY, Namkoong C, et al. Anti-obesity effects of α-lipoic acid mediated by suppression of hypothalamic AMP-activated protein kinase. *Nature Medicine*, 2004;10:727–733.

Ogawa N, Satsu H, Watanabe H, et al. Acetic acid suppresses the increase in disaccharidase activity that occurs during culture of caco-2 cells. *Journal of Nutrition*, 2000;130:507–513.

Velussi M, Cernigoi AM, De Monte AD, et al. Long-term (12 months) treatment with an antioxidant drug (silymarin) is effective on hyperinsulinemia, exogenous insulin need and malondialdehyde levels in cirrhotic diabetic patients. *Journal of Hepatology*, 1997;26:871–879.

Vuksan V, Sievenpiper JL, Koo VYY, et al. American ginseng (*Panax quinquefolius L*) reduces postprandial glycemia in nondiabetic subjects and subjects with type 2 diabetes mellitus. *Archives of Internal Medicine*, 2000;160:1009–1013.

Chapter 12. Dealing with Down Days, Depression, and Bipolar Disorder

Delle Chiaie R, Pancheri P, Scapicchio P. Efficacy and tolerability of oral and intramuscular S-adenosyl-L-methionine 1,4-butanedisulfonate

(SAMe) in the treatment of major depression: comparison with imipramine in 2 multicenter studies. *American Journal of Clinical Nutrition*, 2002;76:1172S–1176S.

Hirashima F, Parow AM, Stoll AL, et al. Omega-3 fatty acid treatment and T2 whole brain relaxation times in bipolar disorder. *American Journal of Psychiatry*, 2004;161:1922–1924.

Mischoulon D, Fava M. Role of S-adenosyl-L-methionine in the treatment of depression: a review of the evidence. *American Journal of Clinical Nutrition*, 2002;76(5):1158S–1161S.

Schrader E. Equivalence of St. John's wort extract (Ze 117) and fluoxetine: a randomized controlled study in mild-moderate depression. *International Clinical Psychopharmacology*, 2000;15:61–68.

Schmidt PJ, Daly RC, Bloch M, et al. Dehydroepiandrosterone monotherapy in midlife-onset major and minor depression. *Archives of General Psychiatry*, 2005;62:154–162.

Stoll AL, Severus E, Freeman MP, et al. Omega-3 fatty acids in bipolar disorder. *Archives of General Psychiatry*, 1999;56:407–412.

Chapter 13. Dealing with Alcohol and Drug Abuse

Kim H, Jhoo W, Shin E, et al. Selenium deficiency potentiates methamphetamine-induced nigral neuronal loss: comparison with MPTP model. *Brain Research*, 2000;862:247–252.

Lafleur DL, Pittenger C, Kelmendi B, et al. N-acetylcysteine augmentation in serotonin reuptake inhibitor refractory obsessive-compulsive disorder. *Psychopharmacology*, 2006;184:254–256.

Lauritzen I, Blondeau, Heurteaux C, et al. Polyunsaturated fatty acids are potent neuroprotectors. *EMBO Journal*, 2000;19:1784–1793.

Pittenger C, Krystal JH, Coric V. Initial evidence of the beneficial effects of glutamate-modulating agents in the treatment of self-injurious behavior associated with borderline personality disorder. *Journal of Clinical Psychiatry*, 2005;66(11):1492–1493.

Sekine Y, Ouchi Y, Takei N, et al. Brain serotonin transporter density and aggression in abstinent methamphetamine abusers. *Archives of General Psychiatry*, 2006;63:90–100.

Virmani A, Gaetani F, Binienda Z. Effects of metabolic modifiers such as carnitines, coenzyme Q10, and PUFAs against different forms of neurotoxic insulins: metabolic inhibitors, MPTP, and methamphetamine. *Annals of the New York Academy of Sciences*, 2005;1053:183–191.

INDEX

abuse. *See* substance abuse
acetylcholine, 45, 69
adrenal glands, 47
adrenaline, 205, 207
Aioli, Easy Pesto, 108
"air rage," 170
alcohol, 201, 215
Alcoholics Anonymous, 241, 242
alphabetic (supplement), 219
alpha-lipoic acid, 219
alpha waves, 78, 179, 182
Alzheimer's disease, 45, 67, 68
amino acids, 44–45, 75–79
AMP-activated protein kinase
    (AMPK), 219
anger disorders, 3, 20, 45, 157,
    167–82
  lifestyle and, 180–82
  psychological tips for dealing with,
    172–75
  supplements for, 61, 63, 64,
    178–80, 188–90
  violent behavior and. *See* violent
    behavior
antidepressants
  folic acid and, 67, 68
  prescription drugs, 40, 62, 80, 89,
    195, 198, 221, 226–27, 230

supplements as, 60, 63, 64, 66, 69,
    70, 71, 72, 73, 74, 78, 79–80,
    83–85, 226, 229–33
antioxidants, 49, 178, 202, 211
anxiety disorders, 3, 20, 183–202
  eating habits and, 185, 186–88,
    196, 201
  lifestyle changes, 190–91
  marketing methods and, 31–32
  psychological tips for, 186
  supplements for, 60, 66, 69, 70, 73,
    76, 77–78, 79–80, 82–83,
    188–90, 193–96, 197–98
Apple Cider Vinaigrette Dressing,
    124
Arnedt, J. Todd, 148–49
aromatherapy, 70
Asparagus, Broiled, 114
aspartame, 49
Atkins, Robert, 75
attention-deficit-hyperactivity disor-
    der (ADHD), 50, 73, 203
  adult behavior resembling, 35–36,
    204–5. See also impulsive and
    distractible behavior
autism, 77, 201
Avocado and Roasted Bell Peppers,
    118

ABOUT THE AUTHOR

Jack Challem, known as The Nutrition Reporter™, is one of America's most trusted health writers, with thirty years of experience describing research on nutrition, vitamins, minerals, and herbs. He graduated with high honors from Northeastern Illinois University and is both a sociologist and a nutrition expert. Challem is the author of *Feed Your Genes Right*, *The Inflammation Syndrome*, and the lead author of the best-selling *Syndrome X: The Complete Nutritional Program to Prevent and Reverse Insulin Resistance*. He is also the series editor for the fifty-volume User's Guide series of health paperback books and the author of several titles in that series. He writes *The Nutrition Reporter*™ newsletter and contributes regularly to many magazines, including *Alternative Medicine, Better Nutrition, Body & Soul, Experience Life, Let's Live*, and others. Jack's scientific articles have appeared in *Free Radical Biology & Medicine, Journal of Orthomolecular Medicine, Medical Hypotheses*, and other journals. In addition, he is a columnist for *Alternative & Complementary Therapies*. Jack is a frequent speaker at nutritional medicine conferences and to consumer health groups.